7/77

For Joel Elkes
with thanks and best wishes,
    Ross Baldessarini

Chemotherapy

in Psychiatry

Chemotherapy in Psychiatry

Ross J. Baldessarini, M.D.

Harvard University Press
Cambridge, Massachusetts
and London, England   1977

Library of Congress Cataloging in Publication Data

Baldessarini, Ross J.   1937–
    Chemotherapy in psychiatry.

    Bibliography: p.
    Includes index.
        1. Psychopharmacology.   I. Title. [DNLM: 1. Mental
disorders—Drug therapy.   2. Psychopharmacology.
QV77 B176c]
RC483.B26   616.8′918   76-30322
ISBN 0-674-11380-2

For Fran, Anne, and John,
who are tolerant and patient,
and in memory of Obie

Preface

This survey of the various categories of psychotropic agents in current clinical use indicates that there are effective and safe medical treatments for most of the major psychiatric illnesses. Their usefulness is most apparent in the more acute and severe forms of psychiatric illness. Unfortunately, many persistent forms of psychosis, neurosis, and character disorder are more poorly responsive to such medical treatments. Even in those syndromes that respond well to medications, the most efficient and humane use of medical therapies in psychiatry, as in general medicine, requires that applied medical technology be balanced with attention to patient and clinician as individuals and members of a social network. Effective application of psychiatric chemotherapy clearly requires more than recognition of a syndrome and selection of an appropriate agent and dose. Personal sensitivity and effective application of more traditional psychological and social aspects of psychiatric care are still required. The limited efficacy and sometimes serious toxicity of most of the available agents indicate the need to develop better drugs—a need existing for many years, as there have been remarkably few fundamentally new agents since the 1950s.

The development of effective chemotherapies has had an

important impact on modern academic and theoretical psychiatry, in addition to an almost revolutionary impact on psychiatric practice. Through the use and study of chemotherapy, psychiatry has again come closer to the mainstream of scientific medicine. Biomedical research in psychiatry, while still disappointing in its practical contributions, has gained a new impetus and new respect since the early 1950s. The careful, critical description and differentiation of clinical syndromes has become increasingly important in the attempt to understand their biology as well as their psychology, and in matching the right treatment to the right patient.

This monograph was developed over several years in a seminar on introductory psychopharmacology for psychiatric residents and in postgraduate seminars in psychiatry and neurology at the Massachusetts General Hospital. In 1969, when the seminars started, there were almost no summaries of this type available, and it was evident that a new textbook would be needed. In the past few years a number of reviews and monographs on various aspects of preclinical and clinical psychopharmacology have appeared. The interest expressed in this book by students and colleagues indicates the continuing need for a brief text to complement larger or more specialized monographs, to summarize a mass of information in this field, and particularly to make clinically useful information available to students and trainees as well as clinicians attempting to keep up with this relatively new and still rapidly developing field.

This work was partially supported by a Career Research Scientist Award from the National Institute of Mental Health (MH-74370), U.S. Public Health Service (NIMH) research grants MH-16674 and MH-25515, and an award from the Scottish Rite Benevolent Foundation. The work was made possible by the research, teaching, and clinical program of the Psychiatric Research Laboratories which were organized by Professor Seymour S. Kety. Portions of the material will be included in a new review of psychiatry edited by Dr. Armand Nicholi. Extraordinarily thoughtful and helpful criticisms were provided by Dr. Patricia Gerborg. Dedicated labor and editorial assistance making possible the finished typescript was provided by Ms. Kate Anderson.

Ross J. Baldessarini, M.D.
Boston, Massachusetts
January 1977

Contents

Tables

Figures

Chemotherapy
in Psychiatry

1. Introduction

Throughout the recorded history of medicine attempts have been made to utilize chemical or medicinal means to modify abnormal behavior and emotional pain. Alcohol and opiates have been used for centuries not only by physicians and healers but also spontaneously for their soothing or mind-altering effects. Stimulant and hallucinogenic plant products have also been a part of folk practices for centuries. More recently, man has applied modern technology, first to "rediscovering" and purifying many natural products, later to synthesizing and manufacturing their active principles or structural variants with desired effects. Throughout the discussion that follows, the classes of chemicals used for their *psychotropic* effects (altering feelings, thinking and behavior) will be referred to by the somewhat awkward terms *antipsychotic, antidepressant* and *antianxiety* agents. This system of terminology grows out of the *allopathic* tradition of modern scientific medicine that treats with drugs producing effects opposite or antagonistic to those of a given illness. It has been estimated that perhaps ten percent of the American population at present use psychotropic medications by prescription.

The modern era of psychopharmacology has been dated from 1949, when the antimanic effects of the lithium ion were discovered, or 1952, when reserpine was isolated and chlorpromazine and the monoamine oxidase inhibitor iproniazid were introduced into Western medicine. Also in the early 1950s, the antidepressant monoamine oxidase (MAO) inhibitors and, soon thereafter, the tricyclic antidepressant agents were introduced. Use of meprobamate began in 1954, and chlordiazepoxide was being developed before 1960. Thus, by the end of the 1950s, psychiatry had available therapeutic agents for the major psychoses—including schizophrenia, mania, and severe depression—and more minor neurotic disorders. Remarkably few new kinds of psychotherapeutic agents have come along since that time. The past twenty years have been marked by an accumulation of structural analogues of the earlier agents, with very similar effects, and by considerable gains in understanding the biological and clinical actions of the drugs and their appropriate use.

The impact of modern psychopharmaceuticals on the practice of psychiatry in the 1950s and 1960s has been compared to the impact of the antibiotics on medicine. Quantitatively, the utilization of chlorpromazine compares well with that of penicillin: in the first decade of its availability this antipsychotic drug was given to approximately fifty million patients throughout the world, and about 10,000 scientific papers were written about it. In the 1970s the tens of millions of prescriptions for psychoactive agents in the United States account for almost twenty percent of all prescriptions, a fact that underscores the revolutionary impact of these drugs on clinical as well as theoretical psychiatry.

Prior to the 1950s, most severely disturbed psychiatric patients were managed in relatively secluded private or public institutions, usually with locked doors, barred windows, and other physical restraints. The few medical means of managing them included the use of barbiturates, bromides, narcotics, and anticholinergic drugs such as scopolamine for sedation; as well as soothing baths and wet packs; "shock" therapies with insulin, atropine, or convulsant drugs, and later electrically induced convulsions; and neurosurgical techniques including prefrontal leucotomy. Since then most of those forms of treatment except for electroconvulsive treatments (ECT) have virtually disappeared; most locked doors have opened; patients, and psychiatric facilities themselves, have been returned to "the community," to general hospitals, and to open day hospitals or to hospital-based and local out-patient clinics. To conclude that modern drugs have been solely responsible for these changes would be a gross exaggeration. In the same period, partly independent changes in the management of psychiatric patients were also beginning; these included the use of group and milieu techniques, an appreciation of the untoward regressive effects of institutions upon behavior, and a strongly increased social consciousness throughout medicine, particularly in community psychiatry. A fair conclusion would be that these social and administrative changes and the new drugs had mutually facilitating and enabling effects, which resulted in a melioristic trend toward hope and change.

Statistics supporting the important impact of the antipsychotic and antidepressant drugs on hospital practice include the observation that in the United States the number of hospitalized psychiatric patients reached a peak of close to 0.6 million in 1955, with an initially rapid, and now slower downward trend (to about 0.2 million in 1974), despite an increase in the total population. This change has resulted not only from beneficial effects of the modern drugs but also from policy decisions to alter the pattern of health-care delivery, including decisions to reduce the number of available beds in many public institutions. Rates of new admissions and of readmissions have not declined apace with the potentially misleading decline in the prevalence of hospitalization; in certain categories, especially among the very young and the very old, new admission rates have increased since the 1950s, and there continues to be a high rate of turnover of hospitalized patients in all categories. Although a number of patients who might formerly have been hospitalized are now kept "in the community," often under conditions of marginal or inadequate adjustment that cause considerable stress to their families, certainly a large proportion of patients formerly kept in hospitals for many months are now capable of returning to useful and productive lives in weeks or even days thanks to the current philosophy of care *and* the effects of modern chemotherapy.

A number of very serious problems remain despite striking improvements in the management of patients with psychoses. Whereas many acute episodes of psychosis can be interrupted or shortened with modern therapies and highly disturbed or regressed behavior is now relatively infrequent even in public mental institutions, available chemotherapies have severe shortcomings. These include limitations of efficacy and problems of toxicity. Many chronic and difficult schizophrenic patients do not respond well to antipsychotic drugs, and the temptation to "do something" by continuing to use these medications indefinitely runs the risk of potentially irreversible neurological toxicity. The antidepressant drugs are not only relatively toxic, potentially lethal, and used in a population at high suicidal risk, but are also slow and clinically unsatisfactory drugs; their efficacy in comparison to placebo has not always been obvious.

The Development of New Agents

Most of the available psychopharmaceuticals have been developed in one of three basic ways: rediscovering and exploiting a folk usage of a natural product, often with the synthesis of similar molecules with comparable effects (for example, reserpine, opioids, amphetamines); serendipitous or accidental observation that an agent developed for another purpose has a desirable but unexpected clinical effect (chlorpromazine, iproniazid, imipramine, meprobamate); or synthesizing and screening structural analogues of known products or entirely novel compounds (piperazine phenothiazines, thioxanthenes, butyrophenones). One important guiding principle that underlies the process of drug development in the psychopharmaceutical industry is the profit motive: psychoactive compounds represent tens of millions of prescriptions and hundreds of millions of dollars annually in this country alone. There is a tendency to rediscover only slightly altered old drugs, owing partly to a desire to break into a highly profitable market and partly to the limited possibility of predicting structure–activity relationships in new molecules.

The current procedure for developing new agents is established by tradition and by the regulations of the U. S. Food and Drug Administration (FDA). Once the potential clinical usefulness of a new molecule is suspected, initial animal experimentation is conducted to establish its spectrum of activities and more importantly to evaluate its toxicity and to gain a preliminary estimate of the *therapeutic index* (ratio of lethal or toxic dose to dose producing a desired effect). Next, the evaluation of the new agent proceeds along several paths: basic pharmacology is studied in pharmaceutical research institutes or in universities, and human studies are initiated, usually by a pharmaceutical company. The first phase of human experimentation (phase I) involves toxicologic studies in normal human volunteers. If these are successful, preliminary clinical trials are begun in selected patients under rigorously supervised conditions (phase II). If the initial trials suggest that an agent has clinically desirable effects and little toxicity, broader clinical trials are permitted under more realistic clinical conditions by a number of cooperating clinical investigators, usually located in public institutions or teaching hospitals (phase III).

If all of these phases are successful, the drug can be licensed for general use.

The preclinical phase of drug development, which involves screening of whole-animal or isolated tissue responses as predictors of clinical activities, has become something of a scientific subspecialty within psychopharmacology. The simplest animal tests entail measurement of vital signs and rating of behavioral or neurological signs (such as activity, sleep, coordination, grooming, reflexes, muscle tone, posture, defecation, simple social interactions, or aggression). More precise tests include objective measurement of selected aspects of behavior (such as electrical or mechanical measurements of locomotion, coordination tests based on the ability to remain on a rod or screen placed at various angles, the occurrence of catalepsy, or the ability to survive various stresses). A number of "indirect" tests involve potentiating or antagonizing effects of relatively familiar, standard test substances (such as classical sedatives, stimulants or neurotoxins); changes in seizure threshold; antagonism of vomiting, stereotyped gnawing, or other movements induced by apomorphine; ability to reverse the syndrome of sedation, hypothermia, hypotension, miosis, and ptosis induced by reserpine, or to potentiate drugs known to reverse this syndrome, such as L-dopa. In addition, a number of conditioning paradigms are commonly applied to the evaluation of potential psychotropic agents: passive or active avoidance or escape behavior, classically conditioned escape behaviors or autonomic responses, instrumental conditioning with positive or negative reinforcement, "experimental neurosis" induced by conflicted or ambiguous contingencies, the orienting or startle response to a novel stimulus. While such tests have usually been developed on the basis of rather obvious, or at least theoretical, relationships between the behavior measured and the clinical effect desired (*modeling*), in fact they are useful to the extent that drugs with known clinical effects produce consistent changes in the tests (*isomorphism*).

Once a new agent is found to have behavioral efficacy in animal screening tests and minimal toxicity in animals or human volunteers, clinical trials must demonstrate or deny the predicted efficacy of the drug. Again, a subdiscipline within psychopharmacology has emerged in the past two decades to manage the design, conduct, and evaluation of drug trials. The rigorous application of certain accepted scientific principles in phase II trials is essential to provide a convincing and objective demonstration of the efficacy of a new drug, and it is also desirable, though not always possible, in phase III. A general appreciation of these principles is necessary for a critical appraisal of this aspect of the literature of clinical psychopharmacology, which is frankly uneven in quality.

The most obvious requirement is that a study have a sufficient number of subjects (N) to permit confidence in the results. Sometimes a large N can work against the investigator if the group under study is very heterogeneous or the condition under study is highly variable over time; the result may be a tendency for the data to "regress to the mean," with a "false negative" (type II, or β-error) interpretation of the results: no specific benefit of a truly effective drug compared with placebo or another drug. (This same phenomenon can also complicate the design and interpretation of metabolic experiments which seek to define unique biological characteristics of a particular diagnostic category of patients.) One way to manage the problem is to utilize a large N with respect to events rather than subjects, to seek an effect more than once in a given subject as by alternating periods of treatment with placebo and active drug when the time course of the changes makes this approach practical. A related problem is that diagnostic heterogeneity can also contribute to falsely negative results, and the problem of obtaining a sufficient number of patients of a clearly defined diagnostic type is often difficult in psychiatry. One practical, though statistically awkward approach has been the development of interhospital collaborative projects such as those coordinated by the National Institute of Mental Health (NIMH) and the Veterans Administration (VA) for the evaluation of antipsychotic and antidepressant drugs. Another important consideration is the natural history of the illness being studied: for example, many acute psychiatric illnesses, especially affective disorders, remit spontaneously within a few months, and beneficial drug effects must be distinguished from spontaneous remissions.

The experimental regimen chosen for a clinical trial should conform to previously established facts concerning the pharmacokinetics, duration and latency of action of the drug under study. For example, it may not be fair, or safe, to compare chlorpromazine and a lithium salt administered in single daily doses. Also, it would not be reasonable to compare imipramine and ECT after a week, because of the latency in effect of the tricyclic antidepressants. In chronically ill populations that may be used in repeated drug trials, it is important to consider the washout time of a previous agent before a new treatment is started (at least several weeks for most phenothiazines). Comparison of equivalent doses of different agents may not be possible until considerable experience with a newer agent has accumulated. For example, early trials of chlorpromazine that used less than 300 mg/day in schizophrenia gave results that were inferior to those of more recent trials employing higher doses. It is also known now that it would not be reasonable to test 300 mg of chlorpromazine against 300 mg of trifluoperazine or against 300 mg of thiothixene (see Table I). A similar consideration is that dose-response curves of many agents tend to be biphasic, with benefit increasing to a maximum followed by diminishing gains or even clinical worsening and toxicity with increasing doses. This problem is particularly evident with the tricyclic antidepressants.

Perhaps the most important development in clinical psycho-pharmacology has been the attempt to exclude or control bias. Bias can enter a clinical drug trial at several levels. There may be bias in the selection and assignment of patients: "sicker" patients may be overly represented in a group predicted to have a "more effective" treatment; even subtler differences may occur in comparisons of a chemotherapy and a psychoso-cial therapy. There may be bias in the taking of drugs: an agent with an unpleasant side effect may appear to be ineffective if patients omit doses. Chemical assay of the concentration, or at least the presence, of a drug in blood or urine represents the only certain means of controlling this artifact. In most careful studies an inert dummy or placebo, identical in appearance to the active drug is included for comparison so as to control for beneficial effects ("placebo effects") not related to the actions of a drug. Unfortunately, even this strategem may not be ade-quate if side effects of the drug make the difference obvious to the patients and the observers. In some cases it is possible to design more elaborate placebos, for example, a barbiturate to produce sedation and a small amount of atropine to produce anticholinergic effects. It is also a good idea to include in each study of a new agent, a drug of proven efficacy for comparison. In most clinical trials it is now routine to arrange the situation so that the evaluators of the patients' responses are uninformed as to the type or dose of medication (a *single blind* design), and ideally, the patient should also be kept unaware (a *double blind* design). The evaluation should be done with one or more of the highly standardized "objective instruments," which usually are rating scales extensively tested to establish their reliability.

Despite all these attempts to control bias and other spurious variables, the power of the placebo effect and the closely re-lated observer bias (patients want to get better and doctors want to cure them) may dominate a study and contribute to either the success or the failure of a drug being tested. These effects are so pervasive that the availability of a new treatment may even affect differential diagnosis. For example, there is evidence that the introduction of the phenothiazines was associated with increased diagnosis of schizophrenia relative to affective psychoses, and the advent of lithium salts reversed this trend. It is also clear that enthusiasm for any drug is greatest soon after its introduction. Since it is difficult in practice to conduct a scientifically impeccable clinical trial, and since even an extremely careful single trial cannot provide compelling evidence of the efficacy of a new product, the accumulation of consistently replicated results in a large number of independent studies is needed.

In the testing of new medications, subtle, but crucial ethical problems may arise. Effective treatments now exist for most of the major psychiatric illnesses, and withholding them for purely scientific or academic reasons is not easily justified. To deal with the ethical problem of adequate treatment, an investigator may forgo the scientific luxury of a control group and make comparisons only between a treatment known to be effective and a newer one of probable, but not proven, efficacy. However, such a design retains the risk of false positive results if the standard drug does not perform as well as expected. Also available is the crossover technique of assigning a patient to more than one treatment, including placebo in sequence, with perhaps several changes made to increase the number of measurable events; this strategy is generally limited in practice to illnesses that remit and relapse rapidly in a matter of days or weeks. It is also possible to start an effective treatment as soon as it is clear that a new treatment is either less effective or slower than a previously established treatment. The increased difficulty and cost imposed by current standards to prove efficacy and disprove toxicity of new drugs has markedly slowed their rate of development, especially in this country. The difficulties and expense of developing new drugs call for increased cooperation among the pharmaceutical industry, federal regulatory agencies, and academic psychopharmacologists because not only has the rate of development of significantly new and better agents slowed in the past decade but also the shortcomings of existing agents (toxicity of antipsychotic agents and ineffectiveness and toxicity of antidepressants) have become increasingly evident.

Summary

The development of modern psychopharmacology has had a striking impact on psychiatry in the second half of the 20th century. There are now available effective and relatively safe medical treatments for most of the major psychiatric disorders. These treatments have had beneficial interactions with changes in the philosophy and administration of health care delivery programs and have contributed to a decreasing importance of prolonged hospitalization. In addition, the development of psychopharmacology has contributed to a heightened awareness of the medical and scientific traditions of psychiatry and encouraged a greater reliance on preclinical and clinical experimental studies of diagnosis, epidemiology, pathophysiology, and treatment, especially of the psychoses and mood disorders. The scientific design and conduct of objective controlled clinical trials of new drugs in psychiatry have become increasingly sophisticated and serve as a model for other medical specialties. An important limitation to the discovery of new agents is that many of the preclinical methods for screening compounds with potentially useful effects have led to the discovery of compounds with previously known effects and toxic actions.

2. Antipsychotic Agents

Antipsychotic agents include a number of compounds proven effective in the management of a broad range of psychotic symptoms and particularly useful in the treatment of schizophrenia and mania. Nearly all of the currently available agents produce a variety of neurological effects in animals and in patients, and there has been considerable speculation that the extrapyramidal effects of these drugs maybe necessary and even desirable. Some psychopharmacologists have been so struck by the regular association between antipsychotic effects and extrapyramidal motor effects that they have suggested the term *neuroleptic* (producing signs of neurological disorder) for this class of drugs, a usage common in Europe. The preclinical screening of new agents in this class has depended almost entirely on the observation of motor effects in animals. Although this manner of developing new agents has had practical advantages, it may have retarded the search for agents that have antipsychotic effects without neurological side effects. The recent description of at least one agent (clozapine) that may have such desirable properties supports the conclusion that the more general and hopeful term *antipsychotic* is to be preferred while the search for drugs lacking neurological toxicity is pursued.

The earliest antipsychotic drugs were the phenothiazines and the *Rauwolfia* alkaloids, notably reserpine, (1952–53), although the usefulness of lithium salts for the management of excited or manic patients had been described earlier (1949). The first antipsychotic phenothiazine, chlorpromazine, was developed by the Rhône-Poulenc Company in France. The phenothiazine nucleus had been synthesized late in the 19th century with the development of such aniline dyes as methylene blue (1876). The history of the study of these dyestuffs is intimately related to the early development by P. Ehrlich and others of the theory of specific drug–tissue interactions—a cornerstone of general pharmacology. Ehrlich even suggested that methylene blue might be of use in treating psychoses in the 1890s. Like several of the thionine dyes, phenothiazine itself was for a time used clinically as an antimicrobial agent. In the late 1930s, a phenothiazine derivative, promethazine (Phenergan) was noted to have antihistaminic and sedative properties by P. Charpentier at the Rhône-Poulenc Laboratories, and it was in the hope of finding molecules with similar properties that chlorpromazine was developed. Antihistaminic sedative agents had been given to agitated psychotic patients in the 1940s, but with little benefit, so that the eventual success of chlorpromazine was quite unexpected. Chlorpromazine was first tried clinically in 1951 as a preanesthetic sedative by the French surgeon, H. Laborit, who described some of its peculiar effects on behavior ("artificial hibernation"); these included retention of consciousness associated with striking indifference to the surroundings. In 1951–52 in Paris, several psychiatrists noted the ability of the new agent to increase the efficacy with which barbiturates sedated manic and other psychotic patients. In 1952–53, J. Delay and P. Deniker reported further experience with the new agent used alone in psychiatric patients in Paris. The drug was given as early as 1954 in the United States, where at first its unique usefulness in psychosis was not appreciated, although it was used as an antiemetic, sedative, and hypothermic agent.

Types of Molecules with Antipsychotic Effects

Nearly 20 phenothiazines have reached the stage of clinical application since the introduction of chlorpromazine (Table 1, Figure 1). The term *phenothiazine* should not be used loosely as a synonym for antipsychotic agent; it refers only to those agents containing a tricyclic nucleus of two benzene rings (*pheno*), joined through a central ring containing a sulfur atom (*thio*) and a nitrogen atom (*azo*), to which is attached a carbon side chain terminating in either a tertiary amine or a cyclic structural analogue of a tertiary amine. There are several subtypes of phenothiazines; they differ in the nature of the side chain. Thus, the terminal amine moiety may have methyl or other substituents with a straight chain of carbon atoms (*aliphatic* or *aminoalkyl* phenothiazines, such as chlorpromazine, promazine and triflupromazine); or it may incorporate the amino nitrogen atom into a cyclic structure, as in the *piperidine* derivatives (such as thioridazine and mesoridazine) and the potent *piperazine* derivatives (such as trifluoperazine, perphenazine, and fluphenazine). Later, the tricyclic core of the molecules was also altered, without loss of antipsychotic effects, first by replacing the nitrogen atom of the central ring with a carbon atom but leaving the sulfur atom. Since this type of molecule was a sulfur-containing (*thio*) structural analogue of xanthene, which contains an oxygen atom in the central ring (not to be confused with the *xanthine* alkaloids, including caffeine and theophylline), the drugs were designated *thioxanthenes* and became the first nonphenothiazine antipsychotic agents. The thioxanthenes also include molecules with side chains of the aliphatic type (e.g., chlorprothixine) and several potent piperazines (e.g., thiothixene). Further experi-

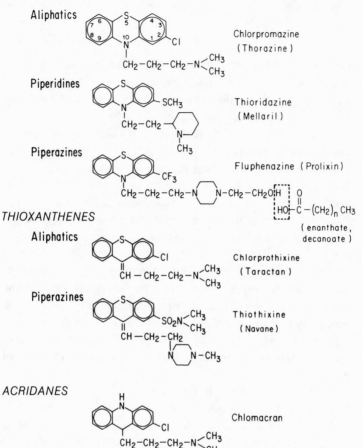

Figure 1. Tricyclic antipsychotic agents.

mentation with the tricyclic structure has resulted in other variants of the phenothiazines, notably the still-experimental acridanes, which are similar to the acridine dyes and have a nitrogen atom in the central ring but no sulfur atom.

The general rules of structure–activity relationships among these tricyclic antipsychotic agents include the requirement for a side chain of three carbon atoms (at position 10) separating the amino nitrogen from the central ring. The addition of an electronegative substituent in position 2 generally increases the efficacy of the molecule, either by counteracting the polarity of the amino portion of the molecule and thus enhancing its passage into the brain, or by contributing a stereochemical bias to the three-dimensional configuration of the molecule. Substitution of a piperazine group for an aliphatic or piperidine moiety on the side chain generally imparts only markedly increased potency (*not* greater clinical efficacy). Higher potency is generally associated with somewhat less tendency to produce sedation and hypotension but an increased incidence of extrapyramidal reactions.

In 1959 P. A. Janssen, in Belgium, while experimenting with derivatives of meperidine (Demerol) in search of a better analgesic, developed the *butyrophenones,* which can also be called *phenylbutylpiperidines* (Figure 2). The only butyrophenone routinely used in the United States as an antipsychotic agent is haloperidol (Haldol). Droperidol (Inapsine) is antipsychotic but is only available as an anesthetic agent although it is sometimes also used in psychiatric emergencies. The butyrophenones share with the piperazine phenothiazines high potency and a strong tendency to affect the extrapyramidal motor system, but haloperidol has much less tendency to produce sedation, hypotension, and anticholinergic effects at ordinarily employed doses.

Several new compounds that are structurally related to the butyrophenones are undergoing clinical study at the present time. They include the *diphenylbutylpiperidines*, such as pimozide, penfluridol and fluspiriline (Figure 2). Pimozide is one of the most potent neuroleptic agents known, and its effects on central catecholamine mechanisms are highly selective for dopamine receptors. Penfluridol and fluspiriline have a prolonged duration of action: on the order of a week, even after oral administration. The only other long-acting antipsychotic agents are long-chain aliphatic fatty-acid esters of fluphenazine, the enanthate or the decanoate (Figure 1). These compounds are useful in the management of chronically psychotic outpatients who are unreliable in taking oral medications, as their effects last from one to four weeks after a depot injection of an oily solution.

Another class of antipsychotic compounds of potentially great importance are the piperazine derivatives of *dibenzazepine* tricyclic molecules (e.g., clozapine, a dibenzodiazepine, Figure 1) or their congeners (the recently released dibenz*oxa*zepine, loxapine which has an oxygen atom instead of a second nitrogen atom in the central ring; and metiapine, a dibenz*othia*zepine with a sulfur atom replacing the same nitrogen atom). Clozapine has particular theoretical and practical importance as it is reported to lack much of the neurological action of other antipsychotic agents (including loxapine and metiapine) in animals and patients. This finding supports the hope that other drugs can be developed to retain desired antipsychotic effects without extrapyramidal reaction.

Other types of molecules with demonstrated antipsychotic effects include indole derivatives (like oxypertine and the recently approved molindone, Figure 2). A large number of other agents have been partially evaluated but are not yet commercially available. Several alkaloids derived originally from the Indian snakeroot plant *Rauwolfia serpentina* and later synthesized, notably reserpine, rescinnamine, and deserpidine, are known to have antipsychotic actions, and for a short while in

BUTYROPHENONES (PHENYLBUTYLPIPERIDINES)

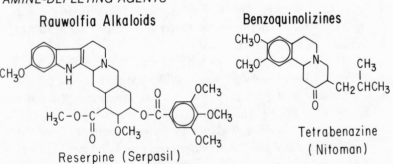

F—◯—C̈—CH₂CH₂CH₂—N◯OH   Haloperidol (Haldol)

DIPHENYLBUTYLPIPERIDINES

Pimozide

Penfluridol

INDOLIC COMPOUNDS

Molindone (Moban)

AMINE-DEPLETING AGENTS

Rauwolfia Alkaloids

Reserpine (Serpasil)

Benzoquinolizines

Tetrabenazine (Nitoman)

Figure 2. Other antipsychotic agents.

the early 1950s there was considerable interest in their clinical effects. A number of entirely synthetic polycyclic compounds, such as *tetrabenazine* (Figure 2) and benzquinamide, share with *Rauwolfia* alkaloids the ability to deplete amine stores from cells containing catecholamines and indoleamines, particularly in the brain. While all of these amine-depleting agents have some antipsychotic efficacy, they have not held up well in controlled comparisons with the phenothiazines. Their limited efficacy; side effects, especially sedation, hypotension and marked cholinergic dominance in the gut; and tendency to induce depression have led to their virtual abandonment for the treatment of psychosis. Although, reserpine had been implicated as a possible contributor to breast cancer, this effect seems unlikely in light of more recent studies. Despite its many limitations, it is worth knowing that reserpine used in much higher doses (5–10 mg/day or more) than customary for the treatment of hypertension can be utilized if side effects or allergic reactions preclude the use of other antipsychotic drugs.

Pharmacology

Despite the clinical availability of antipsychotic drugs for more than two decades, there is a striking dearth of quantitative pharmacological information based on human studies, although a few general principles can be derived from studies in laboratory animals and from the available clinical literature. For example, a careful dose–response relationship has not been worked out for any antipsychotic drug in man. The best available information is derived from a reanalysis of published "success rates" (superior to placebo in overall group response) in studies comparing the antipsychotic effects of chlorpromazine with a placebo. These results suggest that the chance of a study's reporting success was about 60% when less than 300 mg of chlorpromazine was given per day, 80–90% at

Table 1. Equivalent Doses of Commonly Used Antipsychotic Agents, by Chemical Type

Generic Name	Trade Name[a]	Approximate Equivalent Daily Dose (mg)[b]
Phenothiazines		
Aliphatic		
Chlorpromazine	Thorazine, etc. (generic)	100
Triflupromazine	Vesprin	30
Piperidines		
Mesoridazine	Serentil	50
Piperacetazine	Quide	12
Thioridazine	Mellaril	95
Piperazines		
Acetophenazine	Tindal	20
Butaperazine	Repoise	12
Carphenazine	Proketazine	25
Fluphenazine	Prolixin, Permitil	2[c]
Perphenazine	Trilafon	10
Trifluoperazine	Stelazine	5
Thioxanthenes		
Aliphatic		
Chlorprothixene	Taractan	65
Piperazine		
Thiothixene	Navane	5
Dibenzazepines		
Loxapine	Loxitane, Daxolin	15
Clozapine	(Leponex, experimental)	60
Butyrophenones		
Haloperidol	Haldol	2
Diphenylbutylpiperidines		
Pimozide	(Orap, experimental)	0.3–0.5
Penfluridol	(experimental)	2 (1 week dose)[c]
Fluspirilene	(experimental)	—
Indolones		
Molindone	Moban	10
Rauwolfia Alkaloids		
Reserpine	Serpasil, etc. (generic)	1–2

doses of 300–500 mg, and virtually 100% at doses of 500–800 mg or more. The dose–response relationship in man must be very broad since it is usually possible to obtain clinical estimates only of approximately minimum effective doses, whereas maximally effective doses are not known. In recent studies that have compared ordinarily recommended doses (Table 1) of potent antipsychotic agents, such as fluphenazine and haloperidol, with doses more than an order of magnitude higher, it has not been possible to demonstrate consistently appreciable increases in group success rates, particularly when the comparison was extended for two to three months. Recommended doses are thus usually set above minimum effective doses but as low as possible to avoid toxicity. In the attempt to establish an ideal dose there are two important clinical problems: the available methods have not provided quantitative evaluation of partial responses and antipsychotic effects are essentially all-or-none phenomena and not clearly dose related, except in the region of a "threshold" dose. A certain

---

a. Trade names in parentheses are not yet licensed in the U. S. The commercial preparations are available as soluble salts (most are hydrochlorides; Loxitane or Daxolin is a succinate; Repoise is a maleate). Other agents that are not commonly employed now or are less effective are not included, e.g., mepazine (Pacatal), promazine (Sparine), prochlorperazine (Compazine). A recent survey of the cost of antipsychotic agents indicated that the least expensive preparations (less than $20 for a typical one-month supply) were: Permitil < Moban < Thorazine < Stelazine < Prolixin < Taractan < Prolixin decanoate < Repoise.

b. Data are summarized as averages from several sources, some of which vary greatly. These numbers are only an approximate guide, and dosage for each patient must be established by the clinical response. In switching from high doses of one agent to a dissimilar one, it is well to proceed gradually over several days to decrease the risk of side effects from the newly introduced drug.

c. Injectable fluphenazine esters are used in doses of 25–100 mg every 1–4 weeks. Long-lasting diphenylbutylpiperidines can be used once weekly; penfluridol can be used as 2% of a *weekly* dose of chlorpromazine (i.e., 40 mg/week can replace 2100 mg/week of chlorpromazine).

percentage of patients do not respond adequately even to doses equivalent to 1000 mg of chlorpromazine a day, although the occasional unresponsive patient may improve with a higher dose than usual, or with injected medication, or after a delay of several months. The failure rate can also be reduced by the use of liquid oral preparations of antipsychotic drugs to avoid surreptitious disposal of pills. Unique metabolic characteristics of unresponsive patients might account for their failure to respond to antipsychotic medications but have not been described.

Animal studies do not permit estimation of dose–response relationships that allow meaningful predictions of clinical response, but they do reflect what is also known clinically, namely that the therapeutic index (the ratio of a toxic dose to a dose that produces noticeable behavior effects) for most of these agents is extremely high. It is also not possible to ascertain lethal doses, and it is almost impossible to commit suicide with these agents, unless medical assistance is unavailable or there are secondary complications of severe sedation. More than ten grams of chlorpromazine has been ingested acutely by patients who survived.

The metabolism of antipsychotic drugs has been best evaluated in the case of chlorpromazine, although many generalizations apply equally well to other agents. The drugs are rapidly absorbed after oral administration and produce clinical effects within 30 to 60 minutes, and in 10 minutes or less after intramuscular injection. Anticholinergic agents, including antiparkinson drugs, can *decrease* intestinal absorption of antipsychotic drugs, probably by slowing gut motility and allowing local bacterial inactivation to occur. However, it is not clear that such decreased absorption is clinically significant. The agents are highly lipid soluble and have a high affinity for many membranes, including the surface of neurons. There is no impressively regional distribution of antipsychotic drugs in the central nervous system (CNS). They may accumulate in keratin-containing tissues of the body, and chlorpromazine can be found in the skin, cornea, and lens after prolonged exposure to high doses. The antipsychotic agents are known to be only partially excreted each day; a highly variable and unpredictable proportion is retained in lipid and connective-tissue pools, which saturate slowly and undergo slow turnover. Metabolites of chlorpromazine have been detected in the urine many weeks and even months after discontinuation of treatment. These pharmacokinetic facts may contribute to the clinical observations that it takes several days or weeks for optimal antipsychotic action to evolve, whereas relapse after discontinuation of treatment is usually delayed for several months. Moreover, the slow elimination of antipsychotic agents suggests that it is reasonable eventually to administer the drugs only once a day, after tolerance to their acute side effects has been demonstrated, and to include periods without daily intake of drug during prolonged maintenance so as to mobilize stored drug.

The detoxification and inactivation of the antipsychotic drugs occurs largely through oxidation by hepatic microsomal enzymes. Oxidation converts these molecules to more polar, water-soluble metabolites and thus facilitates renal excretion. More than 100 metabolites of chlorpromazine alone have been identified. Most of these (about 80%) result from ring oxidation to form phenolic derivatives at the 3 and 7 positions (Figure 1), and most of these are secondarily conjugated to form sulfates or glucuronides. About 20% of the metabolites are conjugated oxides of the sulfur atom in the 9 position, and less than 10% are dealkylated products of oxidative attack on the side-chain terminal amino group. The major metabolic change of the butyrophenones is a form of oxidative dealkylation that splits the butyl moiety from the piperidine nitrogen. Variable amounts of the metabolites are then excreted in bile and urine.

In addition to the lack of lethality of the antipsychotic drugs, another unique feature of their pharmacology is that they are not particularly addicting. There is no craving for them on withdrawal, partly because they do not produce euphoria. The rebound excitation reported in animals after the abrupt discontinuation of very high prolonged doses of phenothiazines is virtually unknown clinically, with one important exception. Experimental use of ultra-high doses (hundreds of mg/day) of powerful agents, such as fluphenazine, has been associated with a high risk of inducing acute dyskinesias, but not seizures, on withdrawal, if the high doses are suddenly terminated. There is, fortunately, no evidence of tolerance to the main effects of the antipsychotic drugs. There is, however, considerable evidence of tolerance to many of their side effects, including sedation, hypotension, anticholinergic effects, acute dystonic reactions, and even parkinsonism (a fact that seriously challenges the routine use of antiparkinson medications beyond the period of risk in the first two or three months of treatment).

The mechanisms of action of the antipsychotic drugs are only partially known. Moreover, the hope that they would provide important clues to the pathophysiology, let alone the etiology, of psychotic illnesses, particularly schizophrenia, has not so far been realized, although there has been much speculation of this kind in recent years. Some newer observations on the effects of antipsychotic agents as dopamine antagonists are suggestive of pathophysiologic mechanisms underlying their neurological side effects. One important problem that tends to obscure the revelant actions of the antipsychotic agents is that they have a wide variety of effects on many metabolic processes, and particularly on membrane physiology (in many countries chlorpromazine is called Largactil as a reflection of its many actions). Nevertheless, some impressions about their more important actions is emerging.

Information obtained in intact animals indicates that the drugs decrease spontaneous locomotor activity and can even induce catalepsy. "Taming" effects have also been described, and antipsychotic drugs can inhibit sham rage provoked by electrical stimulation of the amygdala. Gross sedation, cortical depression and delirium, loss of unconditioned responses, and deficits of higher cortical function are typical of sedative-hypnotic, or "tranquilizing," agents and general anesthetics; these effects are not found, or are much less prominent, with the antipsychotic agents. As a general rule, conditioned responses are more disrupted than unconditioned responses. Stereotyped behaviors believed to be mediated by forebrain dopaminergic mechanisms, as well as vomiting induced by apomorphine are selectively blocked by most antipsychotic drugs. The local anesthetic actions of these "membranophilic" substances are striking but are probably nonspecific effects observed at relatively high doses. These drugs can also stabilize the membranes of erythrocytes and neurons exposed to physical stresses—but again at relatively high concentrations.

Antipsychotic agents have some effectiveness in antagonizing peripheral adrenergic receptors (particularly alpha-adrenergic receptors in the case of the phenothiazines), and central antinoradrenergic actions may contribute to the sedative and hypotensive actions of the less potent phenothiazines. They have some peripheral anticholinergic (antimuscarinic) action, and it has been proposed that central anticholinergic effects may correlate inversely with the tendency of an agent to induce extrapyramidal effects, particularly parkinsonism, which is commonly treated with anticholinergic agents. For example, clozapine, thioridazine, chlorpromazine, trifluoperazine and other piperazines, and haloperidol produce extrapyramidal effects in increasing order and antimuscarinic effects, which vary by 2000-fold, in decreasing order. Central antidopamine actions of antipsychotic agents (Figure 5) probably have important effects on the basal ganglia, where they block dopamine receptors (and possibly, at higher concentrations, also dopamine release) in the caudate nucleus. It has also been suggested that their ability to block transmission at dopamine synapses located in portions of the limbic forebrain and cortex may contribute to antipsychotic effects. Reports that an inhibitor of catecholamine synthesis, α-methyltyrosine, may potentiate the actions of antipsychotic drugs in some schizophrenics is also consistent with the hypothesis that catecholamine antagonism plays an important role in the action of these drugs.

A number of effects of antipsychotic drugs on the hypothalamus and brainstem have been described; these include decreased release of growth hormone and increased release of prolactin from the pituitary, possibly secondary to blockade of dopamine-mediated control of the hypothalamic releasing factors that control the pituitary. It is not known whether these actions have important adverse effects, but in principle the mammary stimulation would be contraindicated in patients with breast cancer. The antipsychotic drugs block the response of adenylate cyclase to a number of hormones in various target tissues and to dopamine in the brain. The occurrence of poikilothermy as well as hypotension with the phenothiazines may be mediated by hypothalamic effects. The phenomenon of self stimulation through electrodes in the lateral hypothalamus, a possible model for "drive" or "affect," is blocked by antipsychotic drugs. Some evidence suggests that the transfer of sensory information through the reticular formation of the brainstem, and subsequent cortical activation, are selectively inhibited by antipsychotic drugs; in contrast, sedatives can decrease responses not only to peripheral physiologic stimuli but also to direct electrical stimulation of the reticular activating system, while the latter effect is not characteristic of antipsychotic drugs. Antipsychotic drugs have a number of biochemical effects, including interference with energy metabolism at the level of oxidative phosphorylation, either at very high concentrations of the drugs *in vitro* or as an artifact of hypothermia *in vivo*.

In summary, effects of the antipsychotic drugs at the level of the reticular formation, hypothalamus and limbic system appear to correlate well with their observed behavioral and clinical effects, while other effects on the hypothalamus and basal ganglia seem to account for many of the autonomic and neurological side effects of these agents. Many of these local actions are probably mediated by the effects of the drugs on neuronal membranes, but the precise local chemical changes remain obscure.

Clinical Use

One of the most difficult tasks for a physician is choosing from the bewildering variety of antipsychotic compounds now available. The most important generalization that will help to simplify the problem is that antipsychotic drugs are remarkably similar in their main actions and overall antipsychotic efficacy. Available data from controlled clinical trials of many drugs do not yet permit rational selection of a class of agents, much less a particular drug, for a specific type of psychotic patient, nor is there a rational basis for combining different antipsychotic agents. On the other hand, it is reasonable to try various agents serially, in adequate and increasing doses, even to give them by injection, and to persist in giving them for periods of several months, so that a patient who at first responds poorly may have the benefit of any doubt. Moreover, drugs may not all be equally effective for an individual patient, and it is unwise to change to another antipsychotic agent when one drug is producing beneficial results. It is important to realize, however, that a very common reason for apparent failure of treatment is reluctance to take the prescribed medication.

Because there are clear differences in the incidence of side effects with different classes of antipsychotic agents, the selection of a drug can rationally be made on the basis of predicted side effects. Whereas the *potency* (effect per milligram) of antipsychotic agents can vary by more than 100-fold (Table 1), the overall clinical *efficacy*, as determined in controlled comparisons of many cases of schizophrenia, for most agents is remarkably similar provided that adequate doses were used—at least the equivalent of 300–400 mg of chlorpromazine a day. Similar data based on large numbers of systematic comparisons are unfortunately not available for other forms of psychosis, although the same generalization appears clinically to be valid for most types of psychotic illness. There are a few notable exceptions to this rule (Table 2). For example, in about 60% of controlled studies, promazine (Sparine) and mepazine (Pacatal) were not better than a placebo, and reserpine failed to produce results better than placebo in about a third of its trials. Furthermore, since prochlorperazine (Compazine) failed in about 22% of comparisons with a placebo and is associated with a high risk of acute dystonic reactions, it cannot be recommended as an antipsychotic agent. Molindone, in a relatively small number of trials, has not been as consistently effective as other antipsychotic drugs, but its chemical dissimilarity to the phenothiazines is an advantage in cases of dangerous sensitivity reactions; the same advantage is offered by haloperidol, loxapine, and reserpine. Nearly every other antipsychotic agent currently in common use produced better results than placebo in at least 80–90% of comparisons. It is interesting that in 17% of 66 controlled studies, chlorpromazine failed to be more effective than placebo. These results cannot be taken as important evidence against the efficacy of chlorpromazine, since they include a number of older studies utilizing the drug in doses that are now known to be inadequate; moreover, in at least 97 studies that have made direct comparisons of antipsychotic agents in schizophrenia, no agent

Table 2. Frequency With Which Drugs Prove More Effective Than Placebos for Schizophrenia[a]

Agent	Percent of Trials Superior	Number of Trials
Phenothiazines		
Butaperazine	100	4
Carphenazine	100	2
Chlorpromazine	83	66
Fluphenazine	100	15
Mepazine	67	5
Mesoridazine	100	3
Perphenazine	100	5
Prochlorperazine	78	9
Promazine	43	7
Thioridazine	100	7
Trifluoperazine	89	16
Triflupromazine	90	10
Nonphenothiazines		
Chlorprothixene	100	4
Thiothixene	100	2
Haloperidol	100	9
Reserpine	69	29
Phenobarbital	0	3

Source: Appleton and Davis, *Practical Clinical Psychopharmacology,* Medcom Press, New York (© 1973), 35, with permission of The Williams & Wilkins Co.

a. Summary of controlled studies in which the agent produced better results than an inactive placebo at $p \leq 0.05$. Several agents have only been subjected to a few studies, but the indications are that most agents except mepazine, promazine, reserpine, and possibly prochlorperazine, are consistently effective; phenobarbital was ineffective.

was demonstrated to be more effective than chlorpromazine. In a large NIMH-VA cooperative study, 75% of schizophrenic patients given a phenothiazine improved within six weeks and only 5% became clinically worse, while of those given placebo, only 25% were improved, and 50% were unchanged or worse. Ordinary sedatives such as phenobarbital have consistently failed to produce better results with psychotic patients than an inactive placebo.

Clinical folklore based on anecdotal experiences and perhaps on a misinterpretation of the significance of certain side effects has led to the widespread but probably erroneous impression that certain high-potency agents (particularly the piperazine phenothiazines and the butyrophenones) are somehow more "incisive" in their ability to interrupt florid psychotic symptoms, or that the same agents are uniquely beneficial for more withdrawn and apathetic schizophrenics because of putative "activating" effects. Few firm data derived from controlled clinical trials support these concepts. Although there is no scientific basis for these views, there is also no reason *not* to select the more potent antipsychotic agents for floridly psychotic or withdrawn patients. Attempts to tailor therapy to the individual patient's requirements are also reasonable; a different type of agent or higher-than-usual doses may be tried in a hospital setting for *limited* periods of time if little progress has been observed within one month, and certainly within two or three months; and clinical use may be made of the differences in side effects of the various types of drugs. The antipsychotic drugs with low potency (most are phenothiazines) generally have greater sedative side effects and more tendency to produce hypotension in the initial phase of treatment and so are reasonable to select for very agitated and sleepless patients.

The selection of appropriate doses can be guided by the table of therapeutically equivalent doses of antipsychotic agents (Table 1). Most or all of a daily dose may reasonably be given at bedtime to patients with insomnia or those who are troubled by sedation during the day. The practice of giving most of the daily dose at bedtime is safest after an initial period of adaptation to gradually increasing, divided daily doses. The relatively slow clearance rates of the antipsychotic agents make this practice feasible, as well as the occasional omission of doses for several days or, sometimes several weeks, later in the course of prolonged maintenance therapy, without appreciable loss of antipsychotic effect. Prolonged periods without drug are not likely to be tolerated until after at least several months of treatment, possibly in part because the drug gradually saturates tissue pools that turn over slowly, and because the patient's clinical condition is usually unstable early in treatment.

Except possibly with infirm senile patients, it is difficult to demonstrate consistent antipsychotic effects at doses less than the equivalent of 300–400 mg of chlorpromazine a day. Furthermore, in low doses the antipsychotic drugs are not particularly good antianxiety agents and have too much risk of side effects to justify routine use in the management of ordinary or neurotic anxiety. The selectivity of their action by comparison with sedatives and antianxiety agents refutes the older idea that antipsychotic drugs were simply "tranquilizers." Moreover, the ability of antipsychotic drugs to interrupt specific features of psychotic illnesses, including delusions and hallucinations, often with a gradual disappearance of thought disorder, strongly favors abandonment of the terms *tranquilizer* and *major tranquilizer*. Although it has been suggested that they be called *antischizophrenic* agents, this term would misrepresent the fact that the antipsychotic drugs are quite nonspecific in their effect on a number of severe psychiatric illnesses including schizophrenia, mania, agitated psychotic depression, paranoid disorders, involutional and senile psychoses, psychotic reactions to amphetamines, and even some aspects of organic dementia and acute brain syndromes. Moreover, the antipsychotic effects are most readily observed in acute and florid cases of psychotic excitement with considerable anxiety and agitation. It is possible that effects on thinking and social behavior are secondary to reduction of these aspects of psychotic affect. The main clinical consideration is that psychoses should not be treated with sedatives (except for rapid sedation in emergencies) or antianxiety agents, nor should antipsychotic agents ordinarily be used to treat anxiety. The target symptoms that consistently benefit from antipsychotic drugs include combativeness, tension, hyperactivity, hostility, negativism, hallucinations, acute delusions, insomnia, poor self-care, anorexia, and sometimes seclusiveness, whereas improvement in insight, judgement, memory, and orientation is less likely.

In addition to acuteness and excitation, many other predictors of a favorable response to antipsychotic drugs include those features of psychotic illness generally associated with a favorable prognosis or with a favorable response to other forms of treatment. These include lack of an insidious, prolonged onset or a long chronic history; history of a relatively healthy permorbid adjustment and social, educational and professional accomplishment; current episode being the first psychotic breakdown; and prior favorable responses to similar medications or other physical treatments.

In an effort to maximize clinical benefit in minimum time, and to limit the total dose of antipsychotic agents, there have been a few recent uncontrolled trials (only the new treatment was used) of unusually high or rapidly increased doses of antipsychotic agents very early in acute psychoses or acute exacerbations of schizophrenia. Such experimental approaches claim to show promise of interrupting some psychotic illnesses early, sometimes within a few days, and of shortening or even preventing hospitalization, although the first controlled study of this type failed to demonstrate early benefits of high doses of haloperidol. Whether the apparent benefits sometimes reported are due to the rapid induction of antipsychotic effects or sedation is not clear, and this approach requires further study. There has also been a tendency to increase dosages of antipsychotic medications for more prolonged use in the hope that a greater percentage of favorable responses will be obtained. Recent controlled studies indicate that use of hundreds of milligrams of potent antipsychotic agents such as fluphenazine, trifluoperazine, or haloperidol probably does not increase the overall rate of favorable responses. Although a few cases may respond somewhat earlier, the overall effects of doses ten times or more over those usually recommended are similar to ordinary doses at the end of several weeks, particularly with chronic schizophrenic patients.

Early uncontrolled studies also suggested that acute neurological side effects of high doses of antipsychotic drugs were no greater than encountered with ordinary doses, and perhaps even less than usual (the "side effect breakthrough" hypothesis). However, the higher doses are not as innocuous as had been supposed. There is probably an increase in the incidence of acute dystonic reactions with higher doses, and there is a clear increase in other undesirable effects on the central nervous system; these include impressive akinetic and sedative effects that contribute to the apparent worsening of mental status in some cases; and there may also be some increase in hepatic and cardiac toxicity. The consequences of *prolonged* exposure to high doses of these drugs are not known, but there is reason to suspect an association between the total dose and length of exposure and their late neurological toxic effects; thus, caution in the use of unusually high doses of antipsychotic agents must be urged.

To summarize, unusually high doses of antipsychotic medications can be tried temporarily when responses to vigorous treatment with more ordinary doses, say, up to 1500 mg of chlorpromazine or 30 mg of fluphenazine or haloperidol or the equivalent, are unsatisfactory after several weeks. If higher doses do not bring about appreciable benefit within two to three months, they should be reduced or abandoned. Prolonged use of extreme doses is not established as safe and should be avoided, unless a clearly demonstrable effect in an individual patient can be obtained in no other way. The value of very rapid increases to high doses within a matter of hours or in the first few days of an acute psychotic illness has not been established; this approach may interrupt some psychotic illnesses rapidly and reduce the total exposure to medication, but the criteria with which to select patients for such treatment are not yet clear.

There is now abundant evidence that the currently available antipsychotic drugs are effective in treating psychosis. As we have seen, controlled studies utilizing more than 300 mg/day of chlorpromazine or the equivalent of other drugs have consistently demonstrated their efficacy, for the most part in patients within the schizophrenic spectrum of diagnoses. These results have led to the current impression that it is irresponsible not to treat relatively acute exacerbations of psychosis, including chronic forms of schizophrenia, with adequate doses of anti-

Table 3. Rate of Recurrence of Schizophrenia with and without Antipsychotic Agents

Treatment	N^a	Relapsed	Percent Relapsed	Mean Relapse Rate $\pm$ SEM
Antipsychotic agent	1858	370	19.9	$15.4 \pm 0.6\%^b$
Placebo	1337	698	52.2	$55.7 \pm 1.0\%$

Source: J. M. Davis, *Am. J. Psychiatry, 132* (1975), 1239.

a. N = 3195 patients in 22 controlled studies.

b. When statistical analysis of the pooled data assumed that N = 22 studies, then $p < 0.0001$ (a conservative method of computation); when it is assumed that N = 3195 subjects, $p < 10^{-80}$, using statistical methods explained in the source cited.

psychotic medication. There remain the questions of how long to pursue the treatment and whether other forms of treatment add to the likelihood of a favorable outcome. Although there is compelling evidence that antipsychotic drugs prevent recurrent exacerbations of schizophrenia (Table 3), in truly chronic, "poor-prognosis" schizophrenia the benefits of indefinite chemotherapy become increasingly difficult to demonstrate as the duration of illness and treatment increases, and harder to justify in view of the risks involved: particularly the potentially irreversible neurological sequelae, notably tardive dyskinesia and, also, subtle impairment of some higher cortical functions and psychomotor skills. Unfortunately, the best data refer only to relatively short periods of maintenance with the antipsychotic agents; they suggest that there is an appreciable relapse rate following recovery from an acute psychotic illness or an exacerbation of schizophrenia when active medication is discontinued immediately upon discharge from hospital. Interestingly, the rate of relapse seems to change over time: it is unusual within the first few weeks after discontinuation of medication, most likely to occur between the second and twelfth months, and seems to diminish after the second year (Figure 3). For this reason, the usual practice is to continue antipsychotic medications for several months, even a year or longer, after the period of initial improvement. Reasons for this pattern of relapse are obscure but may include the gradual clearance of medication accumulated in the initial weeks of treatment. In management of patients with psychotic illnesses over many years, the conduct of a medication regimen requires considerable clinical judgement and a flexible response to the changing clinical needs of the patient. The safest guideline is to use the least medication for the shortest time necessary to obtain the desired results, with occasional attempts to reduce the dosage or to omit medication for at least a few days, or even weeks or months at a time, and to watch closely for *early* signs of psychotic relapse, a signal that more medication is needed. It is the rare patient who indefinitely requires a rigidly fixed dose of medication.

A more complicated question is whether other forms of treatment contribute importantly to the management of chronic schizophrenic psychoses. Unfortunately, the evaluation of the role of psychotherapies in schizophrenia has been much less rigorous than that of the chemotherapies. However, there is some information based on comparisons of chemotherapy with psychosocial forms of treatment. Research at the Massachusetts Mental Health Center and the extensive studies of P. R. May in California support the conclusion that the presence or absence of an antipsychotic agent made a marked difference in the clinical outcome in schizophrenia, whereas supportive milieu treatment and rehabilitation efforts, or intensive psychotherapy, even when conducted by experienced therapists, contributed very little and were largely ineffective when used without medication. In a similar study of nearly 400 chronic schizophrenics, G. E. Hogarty and his colleagues evaluated the rate of relapse at one year of treatment and found that only 26% of the patients treated with chlorpromazine plus supportive psychotherapy relapsed (and perhaps nearly half of those who relapsed did not take the medication regularly), whereas 63% treated with identical support plus placebo relapsed; the withholding of psychotherapy (drug treatment alone) increased the relapse rates by only another 10% (Figure 3).

The importance of psychotherapy in the treatment of schizophrenia remains a controversial topic, and one that is still heavily influenced by traditions, schools of thought, and practice rather than scientific evaluation. Clearly, psychoanalysis and dynamic psychotherapy have contributed a great deal to our appreciation of the psychotic experience and to hypotheses about the intrapsychic dynamics and possible influences of

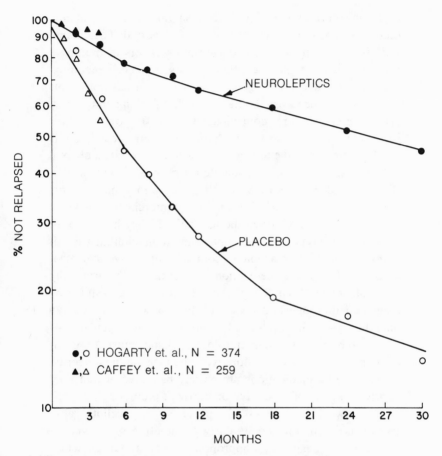

Figure 3. Relapse rates in schizophrenia, the proportion of patients surviving without relapse for up to 30 months. Original data from E. Caffey et al., *J. Chronic Dis.* 17(1964):374; G. Hogarty et al., *Arch. Gen. Psychiatry* 31(1974):603; G. Hogarty and R. Ulrich, *Arch. Gen. Psychiatry* 34(1977):297; and G. Hogarty, personal communication (1976). N represents total sample size, with approximately equal numbers of patients in each treatment group. Note that the rate of relapse appears to diminish after a year of treatment without a neuroleptic drug.

early and current life experiences on the development and course of schizophrenia. Moreover, a few very dedicated analytic therapists have invested enormous efforts in treating a few chronic schizophrenics; their results have been encouraging, but only anecdotal. There seems to be a fair consensus among experienced psychotherapists that probing and uncovering techniques are contraindicated in the treatment of schizophrenia. Psychotherapy alone without medication is rarely attempted at the present time: a confused and incoherent patient is not an optimal candidate for rational verbal psychotherapy, and there is evidence that the antipsychotic agents can facilitate the relationship and verbal interchanges between patient and therapist. Even though their efficacy has not been rigorously demonstrated, on clinical and humanitarian grounds many psychiatrists reasonably combine supportive and rehabilitative efforts with medications in working with chronically psychotic patients. On the other hand, the hypothesis still prevalent that thorough and lasting change in schizophrenia can only be gained by prolonged, intensive, and expensive attempts to bring about characterological change must at present be judged "not proven." Moreover, the idea can no longer be supported that medications are merely palliative or that they deprive patients of a positive or "growth-promoting" experience of "working through" the psychosis in psychotherapy. Psychosis is painful and its early termination or alleviation should be the desired and appropriate goals of management.

A recent source of suspicion about the use of medication in schizophrenia has come from some particularly zealous psychosocially or community-oriented professionals and from certain "antipsychiatrists" critical of the "medical model" of schizophrenia. They have asserted that medications are used by agents (medically trained psychiatrists) of an oppressive society to control eccentric or sensitive persons, and to force upon them a medical label for what is really an idiosyncratic lifestyle or highly personal point of view. Regarding one other unusual set of theories and practices that have become something of a cult, it can be stated categorically that the use of "ortho-molecular" or "megavitamin" treatments of chronic schizophrenia including diets and extraordinary doses of vitamins, minerals or other chemicals, have not been demonstrated to offer anything in scientific studies.

Use of antipsychotic agents in patients at the extremes of the age spectrum raises some special considerations. (The general topics of geriatric and pediatric psychopharmacology are discussed further in the last chapter.) Many elderly patients have psychotic illnesses including senile dementias, psychotic depression, and paranoia. In the treatment of these conditions the antipsychotic agents have a useful place. Although it is common to prescribe somewhat lower doses than for younger adults, a small number of controlled trials suggest that daily doses below 200 to 300 mg of chlorpromazine or the equivalent of another agent are not effectively antipsychotic. There is, however, a marked increase in the incidence of side effects in the elderly, and toxicity limits the doses that can be given.

In the elderly, the low-potency antipsychotic agents tend to induce toxic CNS reactions including confusion, disorientation, and lethargy, or restlessness and agitation. Thioridazine has been popular for older patients, partly because of its lower incidence of extrapyramidal reactions and its possible antidepressant properties. Nevertheless, partly owing to its strong anticholinergic properties, it is particularly likely to induce serious antiparasympathetic side effects, cardiac arrhythmias, and toxic delirium. More potent agents, such as haloperidol, in moderate doses may thus be preferable for older patients, especially when they are used for the treatment of psychotic illnesses marked by agitation, delusions, hallucinations, and hostility. More benign states of agitation that are not associated with psychoses or organic mental syndromes can often be managed with benzodiazepines. Other sedatives, especially barbiturates, must be used cautiously, if at all, due to their tendency to increase confusion, and thus to worsen agitation. Paranoid states in the elderly are particularly difficult to manage with any medication, but again the more potent antipsychotic agents can be tried.

At the other end of the age range, the antipsychotic agents have had their most consistent demonstrations of efficacy and safety in the management of children with gross psychosis or severe behavioral disturbances associated with brain damage. They are not used for neurotic conditions or hyperactivity because of their tendency to impair cognition and the risk of acute and persistent extrapyramidal reactions. The greatest experience has been in the management of adolescent schizophrenics, in whom these drugs relieve psychotic thinking and disturbed (and disturbing) behavior. Doses tend to be twenty to fifty percent of typical adult doses. Dosage is determined partly by the patients' smaller body size, but also seems to reflect both a greater awareness of side effects that impair intellectual and other functions and a basic conservatism in pediatric psychopharmacology. For these reasons, low-potency agents are usually avoided, and the less sedating agents, notably trifluoperazine, fluphenazine, thiothixene, and haloperidol, are preferred. Nevertheless, apart from the question of side effects, most antipsychotic agents in common use are probably about equally effective in childhood psychoses as they are in the adult illnesses.

Toxicity and Side Effects

The most important point to clarify in regard to the toxicity and side effects of the antipsychotic agents is that they are, in general, among the safest drugs available in medicine. This safety in no small measure accounts for their enormous popularity and widespread use. The overall incidence of important side effects is a few percent, although there are regularly occurring effects that are more annoying than dangerous. These include peculiar feelings of heaviness, sluggishness, weakness, or faintness and a variety of mild anticholinergic effects, including dry mouth and blurred vision.

Among the most common side effects characteristic of neuroleptic agents are those involving movements and posture; these presumably are mediated by effects of these antipsychotic agents on the extrapyramidal motor system. For example, the common drug-induced parkinson syndrome may reflect the ability of the antipsychotic agents to block the action of dopamine as a synaptic neurotransmitter in the caudate nucleus, much as spontaneously occurring parkinsonism reflects the degeneration of the dopamine-mediated nigrostriatal pathway from midbrain to the caudate nucleus. Several discrete extrapyramidal syndromes are associated with the use of neuroleptic agents; these include acute dystonias; parkinsonism and motor restlessness (akathisia); late, or tardive, dyskinesia; and unusual reactions, among them withdrawal dyskinesias and catatonia. Except for parkinsonism, the pathophysiologic bases of these reactions are not clear.

The *acute dystonias* occur within the first few days of treatment and are most common with the more potent agents, especially the piperazine phenothiazines, thioxanthenes, and haloperidol. Somewhat more common in younger male patients, they involve moderate to very dramatic and distressing tonic contractions of the branchiomeric musculature of the neck, mouth, and tongue; these contractions may include the axial-postural muscle groups in opisthotonos, and oculogyric crisis may also occur. The main problem with this syndrome is to recognize it and not to ascribe it to a seizure disorder, tetany or tetanus, or, as too commonly happens, to call it hysterical. When the diagnosis is considered, treatment by parenteral injection of an antiparkinson agent (Table 4) can be dramatically effective. Two popular agents are diphenhydramine (Benadryl, 25–50 mg, intramuscularly, or 25 mg intravenously) and benztropine mesylate (Cogentin, 2 mg intravenously), although positive results have also been obtained with agents as dissimilar as sedatives and antianxiety agents such as diazepam (Valium), and stimulants such as caffeine. If dystonic reactions recur frequently, calcium metabolism should be evaluated.

The syndrome of *drug-induced parkinsonism* (sometimes *inappropriately* called "pseudoparkinsonism") is strikingly similar to other forms of the condition, except that tremor is often less prominent, and includes slowed movements (bradykinesia) and rigidity; stooped posture; festinating gait; "mask-like," inexpressive facies; and sometimes drooling. The syndrome usually appears after the first week of treatment and within the first month. Some degree of "tolerance" probably develops to this extrapyramidal effect of the antipsychotic drugs, unlike their antipsychotic effects, inasmuch as the motor signs usually fade away over two or three months, and the requirement for antiparkinson medications decreases.

The proper place of antiparkinson medications in the management of antipsychotic chemotherapy remains somewhat controversial. As a general practice, it is not necessary to use antiparkinson medications "prophylactically" before extrapyramidal side effects develop, although this is sometimes done. It is less reasonable to continue using these agents at constant dosage for longer than two or three months. A number of practical and theoretical reasons support the recommendation to use the lowest possible doses of antiparkinson drugs for the shortest time possible: dystonic crises and severe parkinson reactions are not routinely to be expected; treatment can easily be initiated when it is indicated; tolerance to the early extrapyramidal effects of antipsychotic drugs is usual; and the potent anticholinergic properties of antiparkinson agents can induce toxic brain syndromes, which are not always immediately recognized in psychotic patients. Moreover, there is evidence that anticholinergic agents can diminish the intestinal absorption of antipsychotic medications, and preliminary evidence that they might partially interfere with antipsychotic effectiveness. There is also good evidence that anticholinergic agents can worsen many cases of tardive dyskinesia, and some theoretical reasons to suspect that they might contribute to the risk of developing it. Mild antiparkinson effects can be clinically useful in estimating an effective dosage early in treatment before antipsychotic effects appear. Among the antiparkinson agents, those most widely used to treat drug-induced parkinsonism are the anticholinergic and antihistaminic agents (Table 4). Amantadine (Symmetrel) may also be useful; its actions are obscure, but it has almost no anticholinergic activity and may be less toxic than other antiparkinson agents. Although the dopamine agonists, amphetamines, and a precursor, L-dopa, can be used in spontaneous forms of parkinsonism, their tendency to induce agitation and to exacerbate psychosis contraindicate their use with psychotic patients. It is also possible to avoid or minimize the use of antiparkinson agents by lowering the dosage of the antipsychotic drug, or by changing to one with less potential for inducing extrapyramidal reactions. As a general rule, antipsychotic agents with higher potency induce dystonic reactions and parkinsonism with greater frequency than less potent agents, whereas the less potent agents tend to produce sedation and autonomic effects more frequently. Moreover, agents (notably thioridazine, Mellaril), with low potency and relatively strong central anticholinergic actions are particularly unlikely to induce extrapyramidal effects. If antipsychotic and antiparkinson agents are discontinued simultaneously, parkinson signs may temporarily worsen as the rate of elimination of the neuroleptic agents is usually much slower.

Table 4. Equivalent Doses of Antiparkinson Agents

Generic Name	Trade Name	Usual Dose Range (mg/day)
Amantadine	Symmetrel	100–300
Benztropine	Cogentin	1–6
Biperiden	Akineton	2–6
Diphenhydramine	Benadryl	25–100
Ethopropazine	Parsidol	50
Orphenadrine	Disipal, Norflex	300
Procyclidine	Kemadrin	6–20
Trihexyphenidyl	Artane, etc. (generic)	5–15

These agents are commonly prescribed orally three times a day to provide the total daily adult doses stated above. Benztropine (2 mg) and diphenhydramine (25–50 mg) are commonly used intramuscularly or intravenously to reverse acute dystonic reactions to antipsychotic agents. Amantadine has recently been used to treat drug-induced parkinsonism and catatonia; it is relatively expensive. Diphenhydramine and orphenadrine are antihistaminic and anticholinergic; ethopropazine is a strongly anticholinergic phenothiazine; the other agents are atropine-like. Most are available as soluble hydrochlorides.

The other important early motor symptom that occurs along with parkinsonism, or slightly later, is sometimes highly distressing; it involves motor restlessness, fidgeting, pacing, "restless legs," and a drive to move about and is known as *akathisia* (or acathisia, but *not* "akathesia" or "akisthesia"). This syndrome is frequently dismissed as a sign of increasing psychotic anxiety or agitation and inappropriately treated by increasing the dose of the antipsychotic drug. The reaction can sometimes be managed by reducing the dose of antipsychotic medication or changing to a different agent. Antiparkinson drugs may have a beneficial effect, as do antianxiety agents with muscle-relaxing properties such as diazepam (Valium). Unfortunately, many cases respond poorly to treatment and a clinical decision weighing the distress of the akathisia against the need for antipsychotic medications must be made.

Among the less frequent reactions to antipsychotic agents are *catatonic reactions.* Severe akinetic and catatonic reactions and mutism have been associated with high doses of potent antipsychotic agents such as fluphenazine or haloperidol, particularly in younger patients who previously experienced extrapyramidal reactions including bradykinesia and rigidity. Sometimes acute reactions occur that look more like malignant forms of parkinsonism. The use of intravenous amobarbital (Amytal) is usually not helpful in differentiating this reaction from catatonic schizophrenia, as psychotic thinking may or may not be expressed. The temptation will be to give even higher doses of the offending antipsychotic agent, although improvement usually follows *reduction* of its dosage. There is some evidence that antiparkinson agents including amantadine may also be of value.

Another infrequent reaction is *"withdrawal dyskinesia,"* usually associated with the rapid discontinuation of large doses of potent antipsychotic agents. It has recently become popular to treat schizophrenic patients who respond poorly to the usual oral doses of antipsychotic drugs with parenteral medication or with "megadoses" of potent agents (tens or even hundreds of milligrams of haloperidol, trifluoperazine, or fluphenazine). Somewhat surprisingly, there have been several reports that this practice was not complicated by an impressive increase in the incidence of acute extrapyramidal reactions, although other series of cases include the almost routine occurrence of dystonia early, and parkinson effects and sedation later. Abrupt withdrawal of such doses is very frequently complicated by acute choreoathetotic reactions, similar in appearance to tardive dyskinesia, but lasting usually for only a few days. Similar reactions have been described after abrupt discontinuation of the usual doses of antipsychotic agents in children and young adults. Hypothetically, these reactions might represent a rebound increase in the activity of previously inhibited dopaminergic mechanisms in the basal ganglia. Their occurrence suggests that high doses of potent antipsychotic agents should be decreased or discontinued gradually.

A late appearing extrapyramidal syndrome is leading to a reappraisal of the value of uninterrupted and indefinitely prolonged antipsychotic chemotherapy of chronic psychosis; it is called *tardive* (late) *dyskinesia*. This syndrome was reported in the late 1950s and is now recognized frequently. It consists of involuntary or semivoluntary movements of a choreiform, tic-like nature, sometimes with an athetotic or dystonic component, and classically it involves the tongue, facial, and neck muscles, but it often also affects the extremities, the muscles controlling posture, and, sometimes, those involved in breathing. The earliest sign of tardive dyskinesia may be subtle vermiform movements of the surface of the tongue or the floor of the mouth. Although it is commonly said that an "oral-buccal-masticatory" triad of movements are the most classical form of the syndrome, especially in older patients, it is usual to find abnormalities of posture and at least subtle choreiform movements of the fingers and toes as well. Younger patients often have impressive involvement of the extremities and trunk. There is some evidence that senility or underlying organic brain damage may predispose to this syndrome, and spontaneous pouting, sucking, and tongue-thrusting movements unrelated to exposure to antipsychotic agents are not uncommon in senile brain disease. These are further reasons for using smaller doses of antipsychotic agents in elderly patients. It is now clear that drug-related tardive dyskinesia can occur in otherwise healthy young patients, and even in those who do not have a chronic psychosis. Although subtle forms of the syndrome might be mistaken for the peculiar stereotyped movements seen in some chronic schizophrenics, the movements of tardive dyskinesia are much less voluntary and purposeful and more classically choreoathetotic. The movements in tardive dyskinesia generally become worse on rapid withdrawal of the antipsychotic medication and the worsening can sometimes be avoided by gradual withdrawal; they can be at least temporarily suppressed by administering higher doses of the offending agent or another potent antipsychotic agent, or an amine-depleting agent such as reserpine (Serpasil) and tetrabenazine (Nitoman, an experimental drug in the U.S.A.), or by other antidopamine agents. The currently leading hypothesis is that this syndrome represents overactivity of central dopamine mechanisms, possibly to compensate for prolonged blockade of dopaminergic mechanisms by the antipsychotic drugs. Since the syndrome may be irreversible or may last for many months after withdrawal of the antipsychotic agents, it seems probable that there are other, irreversible neurotoxic effects on central neurons, although the neuropathological information on this question remains equivocal.

It has been said that the syndrome of tardive dyskinesia is more unsightly than subjectively distressing, and that it is usually a relatively trivial matter, but this view is not correct. The syndrome can be embarrassing and distressing, though painless, especially in relatively well-functioning outpatients. In some cases, the patient's skills in feeding and self-care, as well as vocationally important dexterity, can be badly impaired, and severe cases can be as disabling as Huntington's disease. A thorough neurological evaluation of cases of tardive dyskinesia will include a vigorous attempt to exclude other forms of choreiform disease, such as Huntington's disease, rheumatic chorea, Wilson's disease, and other rare toxic or degenerative dyskinetic syndromes. The incidence of the syndrome has varied in epidemiological studies from a few percent to as much as thirty to forty percent of patients "maintained" on antipsychotic medications for many years. It is unusual to develop the syndrome in less than a few months, and there is some evidence that if antipsychotic agents are withdrawn early the signs of tardive dyskinesia may gradually diminish within a period of months. The treatment of tardive dyskinesia is highly unsatisfactory. Antiparkinson agents usually *worsen* tardive dyskinesia. The most effective short-term treatment is to suppress the manifestations of the disorder with potent antipsychotic agents or amine-depleting agents, but this approach usually requires increasing doses of the suppressing agent, fails eventually, and might contribute further to the underlying problem. On the other hand, there is currently no evidence that continued suppression of the symptoms results in their eventual worsening. Perhaps the best means of dealing with the problem, as the search for "non-neuroleptic" antipsychotic agents continues, is to seek to avoid it by the thoughtful and conservative use of antipsychotic medications in low but effective doses, and only as indicated by objectively discernable *and* clinically responsive signs of psychotic disorders of thought, mood or behavior. Some of the reluctance of doctors and patients to reduce or interrupt drug treatment of chronic psychotic disorders can be overcome by the substitution of sustained personal psychological support.

There is some evidence that low-potency phenothiazines may increase the incidence of *seizures* in epileptic patients, although the piperazines and haloperidol may have less tendency to do this. Usually a clinical decision must be made to balance the need for antipsychotic medication against the control of seizures with anticonvulsants, the dosage of which may need to be increased.

Antipsychotic agents have also rarely been associated with severe *"hypothalamic crises,"* marked by hyperthermia, sweating, drooling, tachycardia, dyspnea, seizures and unstable blood pressure. Striking elevations of serum creatine phosphokinase (CPK) may also occur, usually in association with muscle rigidity in a form of the syndrome that resembles "fatal catatonia." Mild forms of hypothalamic crisis may occur in association with acute severe forms of intoxication that resemble parkinsonism. Similar reactions, and rare instances of unexplained "sudden death" (presumably cardiac) have been ascribed to the tricyclic antidepressants as well as to antipsychotic agents.

A remarkable characteristic of antipsychotic agents is that, in contrast to most other central nervous system depressants, their lethality and potential for inducing deep and prolonged coma and respiratory depression are limited. Thus, they have a very high *therapeutic index* (ratio of toxic or lethal dose to effective dose). The lethal dose in man is not known; patients have survived acute ingestions of many grams of these agents, and it is virtually impossible to commit suicide by an acute overdosage of an antipsychotic agent. On the other hand, because ingestions often involve a mixture of poisons, it is essential to consider the presence of potentially more lethal and treatable forms of acute intoxication, including those due to barbiturates or to agents with important central anticholinergic activity, such as tricyclic antidepressants and antiparkinson agents. Dialysis can be used to remove barbiturates; it is not possible to remove antipsychotic agents or antidepressants by dialysis because they bind tightly to proteins and lipids. The central anticholinesterase agent, physostigmine (eserine or Antilirium) can be used to treat the anticholinergic (atropine-like) intoxication syndrome (see Table 15). Physostigmine also has beneficial effects in some cases of intoxication with an antipsychotic agent alone, especially thioridazine or clozapine, which are particularly anticholinergic. Attempts to induce vomiting after overdoses of antipsychotic agents may be unsuccessful because of their antiemetic effects. Moreover, antipsychotic agents may suppress nausea and vomiting due to primary diseases of the brain, such as tumors. One practical implication of the limited acute toxicity and addiction potential of the antipsychotic agents is that large quantities of the drugs can be prescribed with relative impunity, even for patients with impaired judgement and impulse control.

The peripheral *anticholinergic actions* of most antipsychotic agents are modest and usually limited to annoying symptoms, such as dry mouth and blurred vision, although ileus and urinary retention can occur, particularly in older patients. Precipitating an acute attack of glaucoma with any agent having anticholinergic activity is always a worry, but even with antidepressant drugs this event is rare. It is usually associated with "narrow angle" glaucoma, which itself is unusual. Acute glaucoma is an emergency calling for immediate ophthalmologic treatment. Chronic glaucoma can almost always be managed with cholinomimetic eyedrops, even while anticholinergic psychotropic agents are used. Moreover, cholinergic agents can be given in eyedrops (such as pilocarpine nitrate, 1% opthalmic solution) to overcome cycloplegia or in a mouthwash to increase salivation, or orally in daily doses of 5 to 15 mg of neostigmine, or 5 to 10 mg of pilocarpine, to counter side effects of the antipsychotic or antidepressant agents. In general, however, this approach is not impressively effective and is not usually employed, although 75 mg a day of bethanechol (Urecholine) may be helpful.

A number of other *ophthalmologic* problems occur with the antipsychotic agents. The most serious is an irreversible degenerative pigmentary retinopathy caused by large doses of thioridazine (above 900 mg/day). In addition, prolonged high doses of low-potency phenothiazines and thioxanthenes have also been associated with the deposit of drug substances and pigment in the cornea and lens, as well as in the skin. The deposits in the eye can be visualized best with a slitlamp, rarely impair vision, and disappear over many months after withdrawal of the medication. Although penicillamine and other agents have been advocated to hasten the removal of phenothiazines from the eye or skin, there is little evidence that they help. Skin reactions include photosensitivity early in treatment and later a blue-gray discoloration, usually associated with prolonged high doses of chlorpromazine. Maculopapular rashes occur on occasion, and there is some risk of contact dermatitis among nurses handling solutions of antipsychotic agents.

The risk of severe *cardiovascular* toxicity due to antipsychotic agents is not high. Although frank hypotension is not frequently encountered, orthostatic hypotension can be a problem, especially with the less potent phenothiazines and in elderly patients. The hypotensive effects of these agents are quite idiosyncratic and poorly correlated with doses, and thus the ritual of giving small test doses of intramuscular medication is poorly founded. An important practical reason for avoiding large intramuscular doses, especially of the less potent agents, is that they are painful (and may lead to elevated levels of transaminases or lactic dehydrogenase from local necrosis, *not* liver damage). If severe hypotension does develop, it can usually be managed by bed rest, elastic stockings, and elevation of the legs. If a vasoactive agent is required, the rational choice is a purely alpha-adrenergic pressor amine such as metaraminol (Aramine) (rarely will the more potent agent *l*-norepinephrine, Levophed, be required) to reverse the modest alpha-antagonistic effects of phenothiazines; beta-agonistic cardiac stimulants such as epinephrine or isoproterenol (Isuprel) will increase pooling of blood in the splanchnic and peripheral areas and thus worsen the hypotension, and are contraindicated. Antipsychotic agents have an unpredictable effect on blood pressure and may increase the risk of potentially lethal ventricular arrhythmias, partly because they prolong ventricular repolarization. These hazards may be greatest with thioridazine among the antipsychotic agents, but are a much more serious problem with the tricyclic antidepressants. For these reasons, as well as the potential for undesirable drug interactions (see Table 16), it is considered good practice to omit the medication for a day or two prior to electroconvulsive treatment (ECT) with barbiturate anesthesia, and prior to surgery. Haloperidol, the potent piperazine phenothiazines, and molindone may be relatively safe for cardiac patients and less likely to interact badly with digitalis and other cardiovascular and diuretic agents.

Other annoying side effects of antipsychotic agents include presumably *autonomic or hypothalamic effects* such as changes in appetite, weight gain, fluid retention, breast enlargement and engorgement (in males as well as females) and even galactorrhea, changes in libido, and ejaculatory incompetence in males. These effects are most often associated with the less potent phenothiazines and particularly with thioridazine. Thioridazine has even been advocated as an adjunct in the treatment of premature ejaculation.

The sustained prolactin-increasing action of most antipsychotic agents (partly mediated by the antagonism of hypothalamic dopamine) and even small doses of reserpine as used to treat hypertension represents a theoretical risk in patients with an occult or identified carcinoma of the breast. However, there is at present no compelling evidence that antipsychotic agents have a tumor-stimulating effect. Antipsychotic agents can mildly depress testosterone output, but this is of doubtful physiological or psychosexual significance. It had been reported that antipsychotic agents have inhibitory effects on the output of growth hormone, opposite to the releasing action of L-dopa (and many other amino acids), but this effect is also of doubtful physiological importance; antipsychotic drugs are not useful as a treatment of acromegaly, and there is no evidence that antipsychotic agents retard to a clinically important extent the growth and development of psychotic children.

Although there has been a great deal of worry about jaundice and agranulocytosis due to antipsychotic agents, these problems are in fact encountered infrequently. The *jaundice* is almost always an allergic cholestatic type and is usually transient. It was formerly more common than now, particularly in association with chlorpromazine, and it may have become less frequent (incidence not more than 2%) due to the increased purity of the drug. It usually appears within the first month of treatment. Obstructive jaundice can occur with tricyclic antidepressants as well as with the antipsychotic agents. All such drugs can worsen hepatic encephalopathy, partly owing to their actions in the central nervous system, but also owing to their tendency to diminish hepatic function by competition with hepatic microsomal oxidases. Subclinical biliary obstructive effects may be common, as a study of liver biopsies has revealed an incidence of mild obstructive changes in as many as 25% of patients treated with an antipsychotic agent. Frank *agranulocytosis* is rare (incidence less than 0.01%), has a peak incidence within the first two months of treatment, and is particularly observed in older females. Agranulocytosis has almost always been associated with low-potency phenothiazines and thioxanthenes and is virtually unknown with haloperidol, fluphenazine, or thiothixine. Agranulocytosis is a potentially catastrophic and often rapidly developing medical emergency with a high mortality rate. It can rarely be predicted from occasional routine white blood cell counts and *must be suspected* and promptly evaluated in cases of malaise, fever, or sore throat that occur *early* in the course of antipsychotic chemotherapy. Leucocyte counts, frequently repeated in the first two months of treatment may reveal a downward trend predicting agranulocytosis, although early, moderate, nonprogressive reductions in white cell levels are not unusual. For these reasons, some hematologists now advise weekly leucocyte counts for at least eight weeks after initiation of therapy.

A number of defensive rituals of little value have developed in the medical management of patients receiving antipsychotic

Table 5. Artifactual[a] Influences of Psychoactive Agents on Common Laboratory Tests

Test[b]	Antipsychotic Agents	Tricyclic Antidepressants	Benzodiazepines
Alkaline phosphatase (S)	increase	increase	increase
Bilirubin (S,U)	increase	increase	increase
Bromsulfophthalein (BSP) retention (S)	no effect	increase	no effect
Cerebrospinal fluid (CSF) protein	increase	no effect	no effect
Cholesterol (S)	increase	decrease	no effect
Diacetate (U)	increase	no effect	no effect
Fasting blood sugar (FBS)(S)	no effect	inaccurate	no effect
17-hydroxy-steroids (S)	increase	no effect	no effect
Phenylketonuria (PKU) test (U)	positive	no effect	no effect
Protein bound iodine (PBI) (S), radioactive iodine uptake (RAI)	inaccurate	no effect	no effect
Porphyrins (U)	increase	no effect	no effect
Transaminases (SGOT,SGPT)(S)	increase[c]	increase	increase
Uric acid (S,U)	inaccurate	no effect	no effect
Urobilinogen (U)	increase	no effect	no effect

a. The artifacts above refer to *false* positive or negative test results and *not* to actual metabolic abnormalities that can also occur.

b. (S) = serum. (U) = urine.

c. Can also increase transaminase and lactic dehydrogenase (LDH) due to local reaction to intramuscular injections.

agents for prolonged periods; these include occasional routine "liver function tests" and "blood counts," which contribute little other than a false sense of security and possibly some decreased risk of malpractice charges. It is well noted that "liver chemistries" and other clinical laboratory values can occasionally be altered by psychotropic agents as a result of artifacts introduced into the measurements themselves (Table 5). Laboratory tests cannot substitute for an alert and well-informed physician.

The safety of antipsychotic agents in *pregnancy and lactation* has not yet been established. These agents do pass the blood-placenta barrier as well as the blood-brain barrier, and they are to some extent secreted in human milk. They can induce a mild degree of sedation followed by motor excitement in the newborn. There is no evidence that they are responsible for an increased incidence of fetal malformations. Nevertheless, the current consensus is that the use of antipsychotic agents should be avoided as far as possible in pregnancy and lactation, and certainly in the first trimester of pregnancy. On the other hand, clinical judgement must be exercised when the indications for medication or psychiatric hospitalization during pregnancy are compelling.

Elderly patients treated with antipsychotic agents are particularly likely to be troubled by toxic effects of all types, and unwanted effects on the brain and behavior may be most striking. Generally, except for the increased incidence and seriousness of effects in the elderly, the qualitative nature of the side effects of antipsychotic agents does not change with advancing age. Although there is a tendency to keep doses of antipsychotic agents low because of the intolerance of older patients to side effects, daily doses less than the equivalent of 200 or 300 mg of chlorpromazine are usually ineffective in the control of psychotic thought, affect, and behavior. Thus, minimally effective doses of antipsychotic agents are not much less than those estimated for younger adults or adolescents, but the margin of safety is much reduced in the elderly.

Summary

The availability of modern, effective and safe antipsychotic drugs has contributed to an almost revolutionary change in the pattern of delivery of psychiatric care. These agents have supported and reinforced the recent melioristic expectations of hospital and community psychiatry. Most psychotic patients can be managed in open psychiatric hospitals or in general hospitals, and the duration of hospitalization has been markedly reduced. Many psychotic patients can be maintained at home, and many incipient attacks of acute psychosis can be managed by psychiatrists or other physicians without the need for hospitalization. There are many antipsychotic drugs; most are, also, more or less neurotoxic or "neuroleptic." Although there are several chemical types of antipsychotic drugs, they are pharmacologically more similar than different, partly because the method of predicting antipsychotic activity of new agents depends upon their essentially neurological actions in animals. The main shortcoming of the available antipsychotic agents is their regular tendency to produce acute and sometimes long-lasting or even irreversible neurological disorders of the extra-pyramidal motor system. A second shortcoming of antipsychotic drugs is that their efficacy is easiest to demonstrate in patients with the best prognosis; results are more and more disappointing as the duration of chronic psychosis, and particularly "process" schizophrenia, increases. There is reason to hope that better agents may be found to produce antipsychotic effects with minimal neurological toxicity.

3. Lithium Salts

Although antipsychotic drugs are used in the treatment of mania, the lithium ion is a unique agent with considerable selectivity in the treatment of mania. Lithium is greatly inferior to the antipsychotic agents in the treatment of other forms of psychosis, and particularly schizophrenia. It may have beneficial effects on certain acute psychoses, sometimes called "acute schizophrenic reactions," in which an affective or mood disturbance is very prominent, and some of which may represent atypical forms of mania. Lithium salts also have a unique place in the long-term maintenance of patients with a variety of severe, recurrent mood disorders. The differential effectiveness of antipsychotic agents and lithium salts has led to a much needed reawakening of interest in the careful diagnostic differentiation of acute psychoses and to a reconsideration of the tendency in American psychiatry to use the term "schizophrenia," inappropriately, almost as a synonym for "psychosis."

Lithium had previously been used in American medicine for the treatment of gout, because lithium urate is very soluble. Lithium bromide was considered a superior sedative and anticonvulsant in the 19th century. The solubility of lithium urate led J. F. Cade in Australia to give animals a lithium salt to decrease the nephrotoxicity of uric acid, with which he was experimenting, in his search for a connection between purine metabolism and behavior. Serendipitously, he noted that the lithium salt produced a quieting effect in the animals and decided to try lithium clinically as a sedative. In 1949 he reported several striking anecdotes of favorable responses among severely disturbed manic patients. This report led to an intense investigation of the biology and clinical actions of lithium salts in Europe, notably by M. Schou in Denmark in the 1950s and 1960s. The results of several studies led to the early acceptance of lithium in European and English psychiatric practice as a highly effective and safe treatment for manic-depressive illness, both for the treatment of acute mania and for reducing the frequency and severity of recurrent mania and depression. For a number of reasons, lithium salts were not accepted into American practice until 1970. These included strong scepticism among American physicians about the safety of lithium salts, after several cases of severe intoxication and even death were reported in 1949-50 among patients using large, uncontrolled amounts of lithium chloride as a salt substitute, while on a sodium-restricted regimen for cardiac or renal failure. It is now known that sodium restriction and diuresis markedly increase the retention and toxicity of the lithium ion and that lithium salts cannot be used safely in gram quantities without careful monitoring of blood levels. In addition, lithium has a very narrow margin of safety (a low therapeutic index). Another factor contributing to slow development of lithium therapy was the lack of commercial interest in this inexpensive, unpatentable mineral and consequently the lack of industrial support to demonstrate the efficacy and safety of its use. Before lithium was accepted in American psychiatric practice, an overwhelming amount of evidence accumulated to support its usefulness and safety. Experimentation is currently underway to evaluate the possibility that other metal ions might have useful behavioral effects; cesium produces behavioral quieting in animals, and rubidium has many characteristics similar to those of potassium and can produce behavioral stimulation in animals. Rubidium has already been given to man safely and it appears to have some stimulatory or antidepressant activity.

Pharmacology

Lithium is usually administered as 300-mg tablets or capsules of the dibasic carbonate salt, Li_2CO_3 (as the generic substance or as the commercially available preparations Eskalith, Lithane, or Lithonate). A chemical component of the capsules has been associated with false elevations of bromsulfophthalein (BSP retention test), although capsules and tablets are equally effective. Other salts of lithium can also be used but are not commercially available. The carbonate salt is stable, less hygroscopic, and less irritating to the gastrointestinal tract than the chloride salt. Each 300 mg of the carbonate contains 8.12 mEq of Li^+; 1.0 mEq of Li^+ equals 37 mg of the carbonate salt.

Lithium is readily absorbed after oral administration, and injectable forms are not used. It is easily measured by flame-photometric or atomic-absorption techniques used to assay sodium and potassium. Unlike sodium and potassium ions, lithium lacks a strongly preferential distribution across cell membranes, and tends to distribute evenly throughout the total body water space. There is some lag in penetration into the cerebrospinal fluid (CSF), but there is no absolute barrier to its entry into the brain; equilibration between blood and brain is nearly complete within 24 hours. Although assay of lithium concentration in the erythrocyte has been suggested as a superior index of brain levels, this approach has no special advantage for routine clinical practice over the monitoring of serum, plasma (or, experimentally, saliva) levels.

The "metabolism" of lithium ion is almost entirely by renal

excretion. As with sodium, 70–80% of the lithium ion, which readily passes into the glomerular filtrate, is reabsorbed in the proximal renal tubules; although there is further absorption of sodium distally (15–20%), there is almost no absorption of lithium in the distal renal tubules. Because the proximal reabsorption of these two ions is competitive, sodium diuresis and a deficiency of sodium tend to increase the retention of lithium, and hence to *increase* its toxicity. The renal excretion of lithium is maximal within a few hours and then proceeds more slowly over several days. The average half-life of lithium in the body varies with age, from about 18 to 20 hours in young adults to as long as 36 hours in elderly patients. An important feature of the renal excretion of the lithium ion that its rate of removal cannot be increased by the administration of most diuretic agents; similarly, additional sodium input has little effect on the excretion of lithium, while sodium deficiency has a large effect. These physiological facts therefore have important implications for the medical management of toxic overdoses of lithium salts.

The mechanism of action of lithium ion in affective disorders is still not clearly established, although several interesting aspects of its effects have been elucidated. Most attention has been directed to the effects of lithium on electrolyte balance across cell membranes, including those of neurons. Since lithium cannot act as a substrate for the sodium pump, the complete replacement of sodium by lithium will lead to the failure of neuronal membranes to maintain their polarization and to conduct action potentials; however, these effects are not likely to explain the actions of lithium concentrations, on the order of 1.0 mEq/L, encountered clinically. Lithium might help to correct a tendency for intracellular sodium concentration to increase in severe affective disorders, as A. Coppen and D. M. Shaw in England have proposed. The detailed mechanisms by which lithium might thus exert a beneficial or mood-stabilizing effect are not clear. Moreover, the basic concept that the distribution of sodium is abnormal in mania and severe depression is not well established. In the brain, lithium at clinical concentrations can antagonize synaptic transmission mediated by catecholamines (see Figure 6); it inhibits the release of norepinephrine and dopamine and weakly increases the uptake and decreases retention of catecholamine neurotransmitters in presynaptic nerve terminals. Lithium ion also interferes with the ability of several hormones, including the catecholamines, to stimulate adenylate cyclase, which is believed to be an important component of the receptor mechanism of many hormones, including the catecholamines. All of this information accords well with the popular hypothesis that, in mania, catecholamines may be functionally overactive in the brain, but it does not help to explain the reported mood-normalizing actions of the ion in recurrent depressive illnesses. Lithium ion can also bring about subtle and poorly characterized changes in the cellular uptake and oxidation of glucose. A number of other reported effects of high concentrations of lithium ion on behavior and neuronal function probably are not related to its clinical actions.

Clinical Use

In the United States, lithium carbonate was not licensed for the treatment of mania until 1970. Because there is still considerable fear about its toxic potential, it has only gradually been accepted into general psychiatric practice outside teaching centers. A recent estimate is that only about 50,000 patients are receiving this agent, while perhaps a million or more Americans with severe recurrent mood disorders could be so treated. A large number of controlled studies demonstrate the efficacy of lithium carbonate in hypomania and acute mania, with improvement rates typically 70–80% in 10–14 days. Much

Table 6. Rate of Recurrence of Affective Illness with Lithium or Placebo

Treatment	N^a	Relapsed	Percent Relapsed	Mean Relapse Rate $\pm$ SEM (Percent)
Lithium salt	329	117	35.6	31.9 ± 7.2^b
Placebo	330	262	79.4	74.6 ± 6.5

Source: J. M. Davis, *Am. J. Psychiatry, 133* (1976), 1.
a. N = 659 patients in 9 controlled studies.
b. Statistical analysis of the pooled data results in $p < 0.001$ if N assumed to be 9 studies (a conservative method), and $p < 10^{-80}$ if N assumed to be 659 subjects, as explained in Table 3.

Table 7. Rate of Recurrence of the Two Types of Recurrent Affective Illness with Lithium or Placebo

Treatment	Mean Percent Relapsing^a $\pm$ SEM	
	Bipolar Illness	Unipolar Illness
Lithium	25.1 ± 7.6^b	21.4 ± 8.3^b
Placebo	79.8 ± 7.8	73.1 ± 6.0

Source: J. M. Davis, *Am. J. Psychiatry, 133* (1976), 1.
a. Data are mean percent relapses which occurred during treatment with either lithium or a placebo in the 5 available controlled studies. Since the data were variously reported as the "percent of patients relapsing," or as the "percent of episodes occurring" during the two treatments, the absolute number of patients evaluated is not given.
b. When the results are evaluated statistically by a conservative method (Chi-square), assuming that N = 5 controlled studies, $p < 0.01$; by a statistical method that accounts for all individuals in the trials, Davis reported that $p < 10^{-10}$.

of the evidence indicates that this agent also has prophylactic utility in preventing recurrent attacks of mania alone, as well as mania and depression in "bipolar" affective disorders (Tables 6–8). Thus, in a recent review of nine controlled studies of the prophylactic effects of lithium, the overall relapse rate was 79% among 330 patients given a placebo and only 36% among 329 patients maintained on a lithium salt. The initial indication for which lithium carbonate was licensed was the treatment of mania itself, although at present prolonged use of lithium for the prevention of recurrent mania and bipolar disorders is already a widely accepted practice. The evidence for utility of lithium salts in the treatment of "unipolar" recurrent depressive disease is also encouraging, but not yet sufficient to establish this use of lithium in clinical practice. The

Table 8. Rate of Recurrence of Mania or Depression in Bipolar Manic-Depressives with Lithium or Placebo

	Percent of Relapses[a]	
Treatment	Manic (120)	Depressive (63)
Lithium	29.2	36.5
Placebo	70.8	63.5
"Protection Ratio" (Placebo : Lithium)	2.4	1.7

Source: J. M. Davis, *Am. J. Psychiatry, 133* (1976), 1.

a. Data are mean percent of patients relapsing in the manic or depressive phases of bipolar affective illnesses during treatment with lithium or placebo. The results are derived from the only two controlled studies that provided sufficient data to evaluate the differential effects of the treatment on the two phases of the illness. Lithium appears to produce a protective effect against both types of relapse, but the results are too few to permit statistical analysis. It is interesting to note that about two-thirds of all 183 relapses were manic in type regardless of the treatment.

evidence for usefulness of lithium as a primary treatment for depressive illnesses is weak and inconsistent.

One of the problems in evaluating lithium's spectrum of effectiveness in psychiatric illness is the differential diagnosis of the psychoses and the severe mood disorders. Whereas lithium salts are a poor treatment for schizophrenia, they might have beneficial effects in some atypical forms of acute psychosis, particularly "schizoaffective schizophrenia" and dysphoric or paranoid forms of mania, which can be as florid as an acute exacerbation of a schizophrenic illness. There is also a growing impression that on close investigation many cases superficially seeming to represent unipolar recurrent depression, and potentially treatable with lithium, are found to have episodes of moderate euphoria and increased energy, activity and productivity, either spontaneously or in response to antidepressant drugs or ECT.

Even though the usefulness of lithium carbonate in acute mania is solidly based on experimental evidence, in fact, the response to lithium by itself is usually impractically slow. It is usually necessary to add an antipsychotic agent within the first few days of treatment to bring about prompt behavioral control of frank mania, particularly in a general hospital or an open psychiatric unit. The more promising feature of lithium therapy is that it may diminish the rate and severity of recurrences of mood disorders.

Although there is still some hesitation to use lithium therapy, the principles of its use are really quite simple (Table 9). In most cases, the treatment will be started during an episode of acute mania or hypomania. There has been a tendency to avoid initiating treatment in depressed patients, but no evidence supports this hesitancy. If lithium is started mainly for its prophylactic actions in a period of normal mood, or if its use is to be continued indefinitely after an acute attack of mania, two important guidelines should be followed: the *indications* should be *convincing* and the patient should be *reliable* enough to follow the required medical regimen. Thus, infrequent episodes of even severe mania or depression separated by several years, or relatively frequent episodes of milder abnormalities of mood require that clinical judgment balance the inconvenience and risk of the treatment against the indications for it. Very impulsive or suicidal patients are not good candidates for the sustained use of lithium treatment on an outpatient basis, because the acute ingestion of even a few days' supply of lithium carbonate can be highly toxic or even lethal. One advantage of lithium in prophylactic treatment is that many bipolar or recurrently manic patients who are reluctant to be inhibited by antipsychotic agents or to engage in prolonged contact with a psychiatrist or psychotherapist, will accept the almost imperceptible subjective effects of lithium and will comply with medical supervision and blood tests.

When lithium treatment is initiated in hypomania or mania, it is usual to hospitalize the patient, although treatment can sometimes be started on an outpatient basis. The initial medical evaluation should include a physical examination and laboratory tests of renal, electrolyte and thyroid function, fasting blood sugar, complete blood count, and electrocardiogram (EKG). Although lithium has been used safely and successfully in cases of severe cardiovascular and renal disease, these conditions require close monitoring of electrolyte balance and excellent medical consultation. The requirements for repeated laboratory and medical evaluations are not clearly established, but sound practice calls for reevaluation of renal, electrolyte, cardiac, thyroid and general medical status at least once or twice a year.

When the administration of lithium carbonate is started in manic patients, the initial daily intake is usually 600 or 900 mg in divided oral doses. The goal is to increase the dose gradually over several days to attain blood levels above 1.0 mEq/L, ide-

Table 9. Principles of the Use of Lithium Ion

Indications
- Acute hypomanic and manic episodes
- Recurrent manias, bipolar illness, and perhaps depressions

Acute Treatment
- Slow action as plasma Li^+ reaches 1.2–1.6 mEq/L
- Usually add antipsychotic agent during early phase of treatment
- Monitor serum level and watch closely for toxic signs
- Expect toxicity at 2–3 and lethality above 5–7 mEq/L

"Maintenance" Treatment
- May add antidepressants, ECT, or antipsychotics as needed
- Plasma levels 0.8–1.2 mEq/L
- Monitor serum levels infrequently
- Li^+ retention and toxicity increased if Na^+ decreased: with sweating, diarrhea, diuresis (including postpartum diuresis); and on resolution of mania
- Watch skin, thyroid, renal function

ally between 1.2 and 1.6 mEq/L. Although blood levels as high as 2.0 mEq/L have been accepted, this is in general an unnecessarily risky practice. Rapid increases in the dose and blood levels of lithium ion will often produce gastrointestinal distress, which can usually be avoided by increasing the dose *gradually* and administering the medication three or four times a day with, or just after a meal. The final oral dose required to attain the desired blood level varies considerably among individuals: younger and larger patients require larger doses. Typically, daily doses range between 1200 and 3600 mg for manic patients.

The most important principle in the use of lithium is that, unlike every other medication used in psychiatry, the oral dose is not an adequate guideline, and the proper maintenance of *blood concentrations* of the agent is *crucial*. Because of the short half-life of the lithium ion in the body, blood levels vary markedly over the 24-hour cycle. Therefore, doses are divided and blood levels must be assayed according to a strict protocol: the appropriate blood levels are defined as those measured eight to twelve hours after the final dose of the day and prior to the first morning dose. In the first few days of lithium therapy in manic patients, daily and then every-other-day blood assays should be obtained. An antipsychotic drug is usually required in the first week of treatment. ECT is rarely necessary. Once the appropriate dose of lithium carbonate is known, it can be continued until the mania begins to abate when there is a risk of change in the fluid and electrolyte balance, and an increased chance of intoxication with lithium. At this point the dose should be gradually reduced to maintain the blood concentration at about 1.0 mEq/L.

For prophylaxis after discharge from hospital, blood levels of 0.8 to 1.2 mEq/L are adequate and safe. Usually, each patient has a stable requirement for a total daily dose that provides the desired blood level of lithium (typically between 600 and 1500 mg, and most often 900 mg/day), although there is considerable variation among patients. After a few weekly blood assays to establish the appropriate maintenance dose for the individual patient, blood assays can be performed infrequently, perhaps monthly or even less often, with random and unannounced blood samples taken as a check on the reliability of the patient. A method to estimate the required daily dose of lithium that is particularly useful for beginning prolonged treatment of an outpatient during a period of stable mood is to measure the blood level of lithium 24 hours after a test dose of 600 mg of lithium carbonate. There is a logarithmic relationship between the resulting blood level and the required daily dose of lithium salt (Figure 4). After the treatment with lithium is established, there is ordinarily no need to prescribe salt supplements, but the maintenance of *normal sodium* intake and output is important. Patients have been maintained on stable doses of lithium carbonate between episodes of mania and depression for many years without serious problems.

Lithium can be used for geriatric patients with severe, recurrent manic-depressive mood disorders. Whether it is also effective in recurrent mood changes associated with senility is not established. Older patients have a decreased ability to clear and excrete the lithium ion and are less tolerant of it

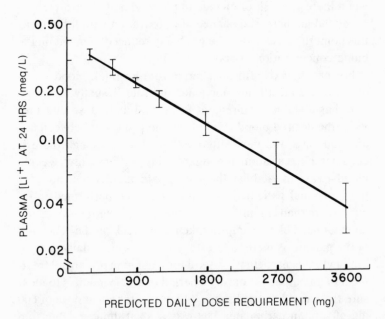

Figure 4. Prediction of approximate total daily dose requirement for lithium carbonate from the plasma lithium level observed 24 hours after a 600 mg oral test dose of the salt. Doses below 600 or above 3600 mg/day are rarely required. Data are from T. B. Cooper et al., *Am. J. Psychiatry* 130(1973):601; and 133(1976):440, with permission.

chemically (higher blood levels) and functionally (greater risk of intoxication). Lithium has also been tried in a number of behavior disorders of childhood, although it is doubtful that the adult form of manic-depressive illness occurs before puberty. Lithium as well as the antipsychotic drugs may be useful in an adolescent syndrome known as the "emotionally unstable character," which is marked by chronic maladaptive behavior and seemingly "endogenous" mood changes, with depressive and euphoric characteristics. Lithium salts have also been tried experimentally, with some encouraging results, in other disorders of children marked by severe behavioral disturbances, with explosive outbursts and excited states, especially in brain-damaged, autistic, or psychotic children. Lithium has no place in the treatment of minimal brain dysfunction ("hyperactivity" syndrome) in children.

Toxicity and Side Effects

The most common problems associated with the use of lithium salts are mild or occasionally distressing nausea, vomiting, and diarrhea, usually when doses are rapidly increased. Effects on the nervous system may also occur, including light-headedness and some confusion, but typically the subjective effects of lithium are minimal and patients rarely complain of feeling "medicated" or mentally dull. A fine resting tremor is common and is of no particular importance, although a clear increase in the tremor or appearance of unsteady handwriting can be an important early clue to incipient intoxication. More severe tremor not associated with acute intoxication occurs occasionally and in some cases has been reported to respond favorably to propranolol.

The most important early means of detecting serious *intoxication* are the clinical signs, and blood assays should only be considered as secondary and confirmatory; when signs of intoxication are observed, the intake of lithium should be decreased or stopped without waiting for results of the blood lithium assay. Early signs of intoxication include increasing tremor, weakness, ataxia, giddiness, drowsiness or excitement, slurred dysphasic speech, blurred vision and tinnitus. More severe intoxication produces increased neuromuscular irritability, increased deep tendon reflexes, and nystagmus; increasing confusion, lethargy, and stupor may lead to frank coma, sometimes with generalized seizures. With ordinary doses of lithium, extrapyramidal reactions are rare, but choreoathetosis or other bizarre dyskinesias can occur with severe intoxication. The electroencephalogram (EEG) ordinarily reveals generalized slowing, with a prominent 4–6 Hz (cycles/second) activity, even without toxic levels of lithium. Toxicity can be expected at blood levels of 2–4 mEq/L, and levels much above 5 mEq/L may be fatal. In acute overdoses of lithium, the usual causes of death are the secondary complications of coma, including pneumonia and shock. A small number of cases of uncertain significance have been reported which raise the question of whether the combination of lithium in high doses with haloperidol may produce severe forms of irreversible and even fatal CNS intoxication, although this combination has been safely used for many years throughout the world and continues to be used. It is particularly important to watch for subtle features of an organic mental syndrome (delirium) in elderly patients receiving prolonged lithium treatment.

In the medical management of acute intoxication with lithium, it is important to discontinue lithium treatment immediately. Usually, gastric lavage, the support of vital functions and electrolyte balance, and careful nursing care in a specialized medical toxicology unit, while awaiting the spontaneous elimination of lithium are sufficient treatment. An important implication of the renal excretion of the lithium ion is that its rate of removal cannot be increased by the administration of most saluretic drugs; the thiazide diuretics or spironolactone by preferential removal of sodium may even increase the retention and toxicity of lithium. There is little evidence that intravenously administered solutions of sodium chloride appreciably increase the removal of lithium, but the management of lithium intoxication should include normal availability of sodium; the administration of sodium bicarbonate is also helpful. Fluid loading; solute-induced diuresis, as with mannitol; and theophylline can all contribute to some increased renal excretion of lithium in cases of intoxication, and dialysis techniques are very effective in serious overdosage. The use of lithium in patients with salt restriction or sodium wasting requires extra caution in monitoring blood levels of lithium and avoiding intoxication.

Cardiovascular problems are unusual in patients given controlled quantities of lithium salts. Hypotension and arrhythmias are rare, although electrocardiographic (EKG) changes can occur. At doses that are likely to be encountered clinically, the most typical changes are similar to those associated with *hypo*kalemia, even though blood levels of potassium are almost always normal. These changes include flattening and even inversion of the T waves; the effects are dose dependent and reversible. In experimental animals extraordinarily high concentrations of lithium (above 10 mEq/L, levels unlikely to be encountered clinically) have been reported to produce changes resembling those of hyperkalemia: high, peaked T waves; T-wave inversions; depressed S-T segment; widened QRS complex; and evidence of atrioventricular dissociation and conduction blockade. Depressed or absent P waves, atrial fibrillation, and standstill with independent ventricular responses also occur.

Severe *renal* tubular damage due to lithium had been a concern, mainly because pathologic changes in the kidney of uncertain significance were reported in early cases of gross overdosage with lithium chloride given to patients with pre-existing circulatory and renal disease. Similarly, reports of renal tubular damage in the rat are hard to relate to the clinical use of lithium in psychiatry, inasmuch as these studies have used toxic doses of lithium salts. A more likely clinical problem is a form of nephrogenic diabetes insipidus manifested by the intake of many liters of water per day and the output of huge quantities of very dilute urine. This syndrome is now believed to result from the ability of lithium ion to interfere with the activity of antidiuretic hormone (ADH) on the renal tubules, either by preventing its access to the appropriate membrane site or by blocking the response of an ADH-sensitive adenylate cyclase. This syndrome is usually managed conservatively by reducing or completely discontinuing the intake of lithium as soon as possible, and it is almost always reversible. It often responds paradoxically to thiazide diuretics, as do other forms of nephrogenic diabetes insipidus, and when there are compelling indications to continue the use of lithium, this treatment might be considered after appropriate medical consultation.

Another metabolic abnormality is the development of *goiter* in patients receiving ordinary doses of lithium salts for prolonged periods. The patients develop a form of benign diffuse nontoxic goiter. They almost always remain euthyroid or slightly hypothyroid, although there may be an increase in the circulating levels of thyroid stimulating hormone (TSH). There is experimental evidence for the ability of lithium to interfere with thyroid metabolism at several points, including the iodination and release of iodinated tyrosine, and some evidence of its interference with the actions of thyroxin on target tissues, much as the actions of ADH seem to be impaired. Again, there is no serious danger from the goiter, but judgment must be exercised, with the help of endocrinologic consultation, whether to continue the treatment with lithium. Rarely will significant functional hypothyroidism or frank myxedema occur, although in many cases treatment with thyroxin leads to regression of the goiter and permits maintenance of a euthyroid status while lithium therapy is pursued. (Lithium has even been suggested as treatment for hyperthyroidism and excesses of ADH.) Other toxic effects of lithium include the occasional development of localized edema, eruptions (especially a reversible, but potentially recurrent form of folliculitis that resembles keratosis pilaris), or even ulcerations of the *skin*. An antihistaminic agent may be helpful for the rashes, and for the rare skin ulcers, topical steroids are useful. Hepatic and bone marrow toxicity are rarely associated with lithium therapy. Although it is not unusual to observe a mild elevation of the peripheral leucocyte count, its significance is uncertain. Lithium has been reported to worsen myasthenia gravis in rare instances.

A great deal of concern surrounds the use of lithium in *pregnancy and lactation,* partly because studies in classical embryology revealed grossly teratogenic effects of very high concentrations, and more recent evidence in experimental animals indicates that very high doses of lithium are associated with fetal wastage and anomalies of the central nervous system. There are also reports of uncertain significance that lithium can alter the metabolism of the rat testis, as well as the motility of human sperm. Together with other alterations in fluid and electrolyte metabolism in pregnancy, there is an increased clearance of lithium; with the diuresis after delivery there may be an increased *retention* of lithium and consequently an increased risk of intoxication. Fetal distress may occur when lithium is used near term, and there may be hypotonia, listlessness, lethargy, cyanosis, decreased suck response and Moro reflex in the newborn infants of mothers taking lithium. In nursing mothers, breast milk lithium concentration is about 30–50% of the mother's blood level. A small number of reports associated human fetal anomalies with the use of lithium in pregnancy, and suggest that the rate of such occurrence may be increased over that expected in the general population. A reasonable position at the present time is that there is enough circumstantial evidence about the potential fetal toxicity of lithium to urge avoidance of its use in the early months of pregnancy, to advise caution and discontinuation of lithium before term, and to permit the use of lithium in pregnancy only for the most urgent indications. All experiences with lithium in pregnancy should be reported to the research registry established for this purpose at Langley Porter Psychiatric Institute in San Francisco.

Summary

Lithium ion provides a useful and specific form of chemotherapy for manic and hypomanic episodes. Its clinical actions may be delayed for a week or more; so the use of an antipsychotic agent may be required in the initial period to control the behavior of very disturbed patients. The main limitation of lithium is its narrow therapeutic index and requirement for close medical supervision. The most promising aspect of the use of lithium is its prophylactic effect in reducing the frequency and severity of manic and depressive attacks in manic-depressive illness.

4. Antidepressant Agents

The physical treatment of severe depression prior to the 1950s included the use of various "shock" treatments, notably hypoglycemia induced by large doses of insulin, and convulsive treatments based on the use of chemicals (camphor and later the inhaled convulsant gases such as flurothyl, Indoklon) or electrical currents applied directly to the head (electroconvulsive treatment, ECT). Of these, all but ECT are now largely of historical interest and have been replaced by the modern antidepressant chemotherapies. ECT still has an important place in modern medical therapies of major psychiatric disorders, despite an undeservedly poor reputation owing to its inconvenience, risks of side effects and physical trauma, and its overly enthusiastic application to conditions in which its effectiveness is minimal and its use unjustified. As currently practiced, modern ECT is not only safe, but also extremely effective in severe depressions—in fact, consistently more effective than any antidepressant chemical treatment. Modifications in technique have reduced most of the untoward effects of ECT, with little if any loss in efficacy, and have added only slight additional risks due to anesthesia and neuromuscular blockade. Ultrashort acting barbiturates used for anesthesia and paralyzing doses of succinylcholine eliminate orthopedic damage from seizures (except in the jaw, where local electrical stimulation can still produce strong contractions). Application of the electrodes over the nondominant cerebral hemisphere reduces postictal confusion. ECT is still the treatment of choice in certain patients with severe retarded or agitated depressions, with striking insomnia, withdrawal, and weight loss, or who are severely suicidal, and for whom ECT may be lifesaving. It is the best choice when therapeutic doses of tricyclic antidepressant agents for several weeks prove to be ineffective. Because there are few absolute contraindications to ECT, short of increased intracranial pressure, it can be a safe form of treatment in patients at high risk of toxicity from antidepressant chemicals (especially the elderly, those with severe cardiovascular disease, and pregnant women). Moreover, ECT still has a place in the treatment of manic or catatonic patients or others with atypical psychoses marked by profound agitation or mood change, and ECT is worth trying for chronic schizophrenics who respond poorly to antipsychotic medications.

Before the 1950s, the medical treatment of depression employed the stimulant amphetamines for psychomotor retardation and barbiturates for agitation. Although stimulants are still occasionally used for mild, short-lasting neurotic depression, there is little reason to use these drugs in most cases of depression. Their use in severe depression is not indicated, and may even worsen agitation and psychosis.

In the late 1940s, it was discovered that several structural analogues of nicotinic acid had bacteriostatic properties and were particularly useful in the treatment of tuberculosis. The hydrazine derivative of isonicotinic acid, or isoniazid (INH), is still used for this purpose. *Isoniazid* and more importantly its isopropyl analogue, *iproniazid* (Marsilid), were found to have euphoriant or mood-elevating and behaviorally activating properties in some tuberculous patients. In 1952 iproniazid was reported by I. Selikoff, J. Delay, and their collaborators in

Europe to have useful antidepressant properties in psychiatric patients. Iproniazid was discovered to be a potent and irreversible inhibitor of the amine-catabolizing enzyme, monoamine oxidase (MAO). Since that time other hydrazine compounds and nonhydrazines with MAO-inhibiting properties have been introduced into psychiatric practice and will be discussed below. A few years later the second important, and now dominant, class of *tricyclic antidepressant* compounds was introduced.

These "tricyclic" compounds have two benzene rings joined through a central seven-member ring (Figure 5). The first compound of this class was imipramine (originally Tofranil, but now available under several trade names and as a generic compound), a *dibenzazepine*. Compounds of this type contain two benzene rings linked through a central nitrogen (azo)-containing seven-membered central ring and are not to be confused with the benzo*diaz*epines, which are sedative-antianxiety agents of quite a different structure (see Figures 4, 5, and 9). Later, structural analogues of the dibenzazepines were developed, among them the dibenzo*cyclohepta*dienes with three all-carbon rings (for example, amitriptyline), and more recently, the dibenzo*x*epines (for example, doxepin), with an oxygen atom in the central ring. The original compound of this class, imipramine, was found in the 1950s to have behavioral effects on animals resembling those of the phenothiazines; imipramine and a structurally related group of agents had been known since the 1940s to have antihistaminic and sedative properties, as well as considerable anticholinergic activity. Because many of these properties and the general structure of imipramine were superficially similar to those of the phenothiazines, a prediction was made that imipramine might have antipsychotic properties. In one of the initial clinical trials of the new drug, R. Kuhn in Switzerland found in 1957–58 that it had little antipsychotic efficacy but seemed to

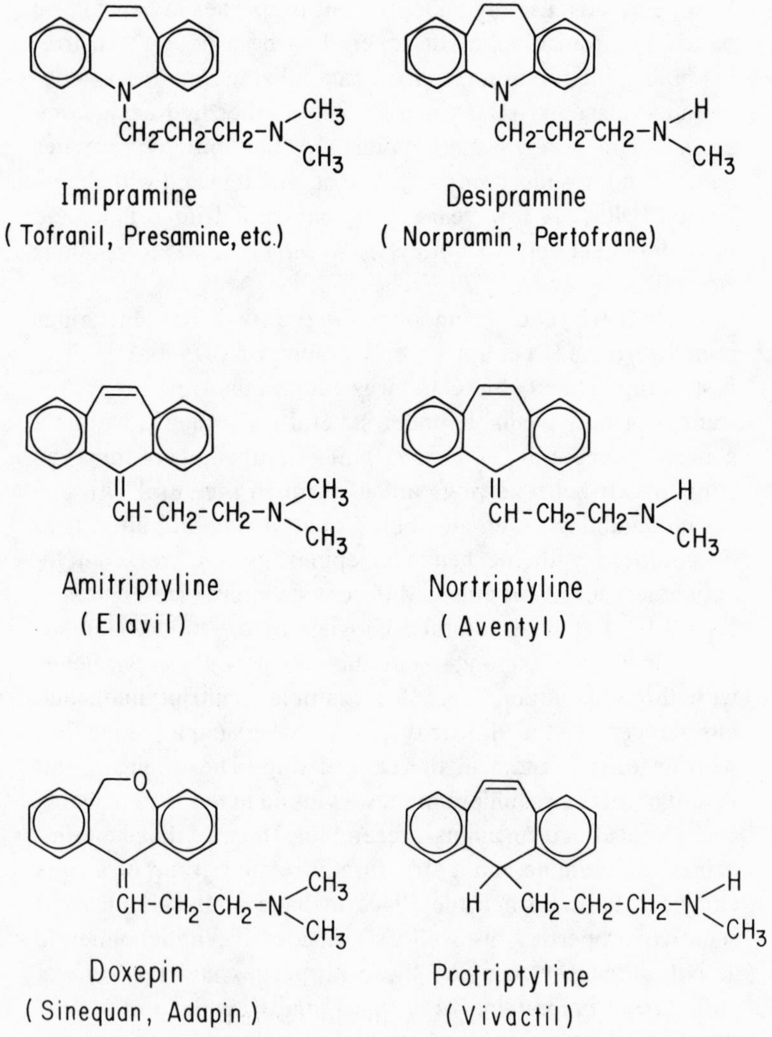
N
CH2-CH2-CH2-N
CH3
CH3
Imipramine
(Tofranil, Presamine, etc.)
N
CH2-CH2-CH2-N
H
CH3
Desipramine
(Norpramin, Pertofrane)
CH-CH2-CH2-N
CH3
CH3
Amitriptyline
(Elavil)
CH-CH2-CH2-N
H
CH3
Nortriptyline
(Aventyl)
O
CH-CH2-CH2-N
CH3
CH3
Doxepin
(Sinequan, Adapin)
H
CH2-CH2-CH2-N
H
CH3
Protriptyline
(Vivactil)

Figure 5. Tricyclic antidepressants.

have mood-elevating and behavior-activating properties. Since that time, imipramine and the structurally related tricyclic agents have been repeatedly demonstrated in controlled comparisons with a placebo or a stimulant to be effective in several types of depression. Although these clinical effects have not always been easily demonstrated (see Table 11), in contrast to most trials of the antipsychotic agents (Table 2), and despite the considerable toxicity and side effects of this class of drugs, they have become by far the most popular and common medical treatment for depressions of all kinds, and particularly severe depressions.

Pharmacology

Initially, it was believed that the tricyclic antidepressants and the phenothiazines were structurally and pharmacologically very similar. The fact that the tricyclic antidepressants have acute sedative effects in animals points out one of the important problems that has limited the development of effective new antidepressants. In the case of the MAO inhibitors and imipramine, their identification as antidepressants depended on fortuitous findings in clinical experiments, findings not predicted by preclinical screening. Since the 1950s, attempts to improve prediction of antidepressant activity in new compounds have had limited success. Some sophisticated forms of self-stimulatory behavior electrically induced with intracerebral electrodes and responses in certain conditioning paradigms have shown promise, but they are relatively expensive and complicated for routine pharmaceutical screening tests. More often, the behavioral interactions of new agents with reserpine or tetrabenazine, amine-depleting agents, or their cardiovascular interactions with various pressor amines have been utilized as relatively simple and inexpensive predictive tests or "models" of the clinical condition for which treatment is being sought. These tests are based on the observations that most stimulants and antidepressant agents have some ability to reverse or to modify behavioral sedation induced by reserpine or by tetrabenazine. These and other amine-depleting agents (such as alpha-methyldopa, Aldomet) are themselves sometimes associated with clinical depression in susceptible patients. Furthermore, the tricyclic agents enhance the actions of direct sympathomimetic agents, notably norepinephrine, and block the effects of many indirectly sympathomimetic agents such as tyramine, whereas the MAO-inhibitors enhance the actions of both types of sympathomimetic amines.

These pharmacological observations and their interpretation have given the most important support to the "amine hypothesis of affective disorders" which suggests that depression is associated with a relative lack of activity of certain amine neurotransmitters in the brain, most probably the catecholamines norepinephrine and dopamine, while mania may be an expression of overactivity of these amines. Furthermore, other amines including acetylcholine and perhaps serotonin may modify the effects of altered catecholamine neurotransmission.

How MAO inhibitors and tricyclic antidepressants interact with the sympathomimetic and behaviorally activating amines can be summarized and interpreted as follows (Figure 6). The MAO inhibitors block inactivation of direct and indirect pressor amines by the catabolic enzyme MAO and so potentiate their actions. Reserpine acts by blocking the intraneuronal storage of biogenic amines in sympathetic nerves and the central nervous system; thus it interferes with the protection of these amines and allows their enhanced destruction by MAO—an effect that can be reversed by MAO-inhibitors. The tricyclic agents block *neuronal uptake* of amines into the presynaptic nerve ending; uptake is crucial for *inactivation* of *direct* sympathomimetic amines such as norepinephrine and

for the *activity* of *indirect*, or catecholamine-releasing, sympathomimetic amines such as tyramine, which must first enter
the sympathetic nerve endings to act. The tricyclic agents also
weakly inhibit MAO. Their main effect—inhibiting the uptake
of endogenous sympathomimetic amines—is sufficient to increase the functional activity of the amines that are synthesized and available to synapses in the presence of reserpine,
and thus probably explains their ability to reverse reserpine's
behavioral actions and hypotensive effect. While these pharmacologic effects and the amine hypothesis of depression have
had an important intellectual impact on biological psychiatry,
their mutually reinforcing influences may have contributed
to rediscovery of agents with similar actions, and corre-
spondingly similar limitations and toxicity. In other words, the
very attractiveness of an hypothesis explaining the actions of
these agents may have retarded the search for other pharmacological actions that might be associated with clinical antidepressant effects. Similarly, tests for antidopamine effects have
encouraged the rediscovery of antipsychotic agents that also
have strong, but probably not essential, actions on the extrapyramidal nervous system.

An important characteristic of tricyclic antidepressants, one
that separates them from the phenothiazine and thioxanthene
tricyclic antipsychotic agents, is that the seven-member central ring of the antidepressant agents distorts the shape of the
molecules. Whereas most of the tricyclic antipsychotic agents,
including, as well, even the newer tricyclic antipsychotic piperazines such as clozapine and loxapine (Figure 1), are flat or
planar molecules, the antidepressants are twisted and do not
lie in one plane. This nonplanar stereochemical conformation
evidently imparts to some molecules a selectivity for the presynaptic site at which amines are taken up by neurons. In contrast, the antipsychotic tricyclic molecules have their most important actions at synaptic membrane sites where the release

and postsynaptic actions of amine neurotransmitters are regulated (see Figure 6). Thus, this small structural change causes a virtual reversal of the main pharmacological actions of the drugs, making them sympathomimetic, mood-elevating and behavior-activating, rather than catecholamine-antagonizing, neuroleptic, antipsychotic, and centrally depressant. Another important difference in the nonplanar tricyclic compounds is that they are more potent *anticholinergic* agents than their antipsychotic analogues, the phenothiazines and thioxanthenes. This central anticholinergic effect may contribute to their antidepressant actions, although that is not certain. Another analogous compound, the tricyclic antipsychotic drug clozapine, is structurally similar to the antidepressants (compare Figures 1 and 5). Clozapine has antipsychotic actions with very little acute effect on the extrapyramidal motor system and has much stronger anticholinergic actions than most antipsychotic agents. However, another recently licensed nonplanar tricyclic

---

Figure 6. Schematic diagrams of central catecholamine-mediated synapses, where many psychopharmaceuticals have important actions. *Upper:* Norepinephrine synapse. *Lower:* Dopamine synapse. *Antipsychotic agents* block release of DA and DA receptors in the limbic system (antipsychotic effect?) and corpus striatum (extrapyramidal effects?) and have some antagonistic effects at NE receptors (sedation?); reserpine blocks intraneuronal storage. Tricyclic *antidepressants* mainly block uptake of amines and reuptake of NE; MAO inhibitors block inactivation of many amines. *Lithium salts* block release of NE and DA and possibly also block NE receptors. *Stimulants* increase release of NE and DA, block their reuptake, and have a weak anti-MAO effect.

Abbreviations: DA (dopamine), NE (norepinephrine), COMT (catechol-*O*-methyltransferase), Dopa (dihydroxyphenylalanine), MAO (monoamine oxidase), HVA (homovanillic acid), VMA (vanillylmandelic acid), MHPG (3-methoxy-4-hydroxy-phenylethyleneglycol), NM (normetanephrine), SAM (*S*-adenosyl-L-methionine).

PRESYNAPTIC NEURON

POSTSYNAPTIC NEURON

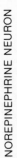

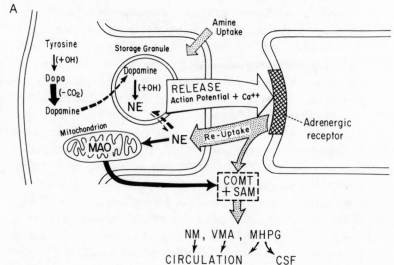

A

NOREPINEPHRINE NEURON

Tyrosine
↓(+OH)
Dopa
↓(−CO₂)
Dopamine

Storage Granule

Dopamine
(+OH)
NE

RELEASE
Action Potential + Ca⁺⁺

Amine
Uptake

Mitochondrion
MAO

NE

Re-Uptake

Adrenergic
receptor

COMT
+ SAM

NM, VMA , MHPG

CIRCULATION ↘ CSF

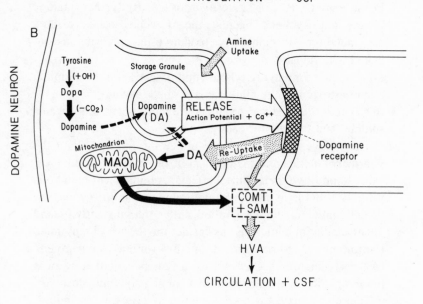

B

DOPAMINE NEURON

Tyrosine
↓(+OH)
Dopa
↓(−CO₂)
Dopamine

Storage Granule

Dopamine
(DA)

RELEASE
Action Potential + Ca⁺⁺

Amine
Uptake

Mitochondrion
MAO

DA

Re-Uptake

Dopamine
receptor

COMT
+ SAM

HVA

CIRCULATION + CSF

antipsychotic, loxapine, does produce acute neurological effects (Figure 1).

Tricyclic antidepressants share a number of other pharmacological similarities with the phenothiazines. They are rapidly absorbed after oral administration. Although several of them, including imipramine and amitriptyline, are available in injectable form for use in patients who refuse oral medications, injection does not appreciably increase their speed or efficacy of action. Their elimination, like that of the antipsychotic agents, is multiphasic. About half is rapidly eliminated—two-thirds of this in the urine and one-third in the feces—within two or three days, but that fraction remaining more firmly bound to plasma and tissue protein undergoes slower excretion over several weeks. A practical consequence of the affinity of the antidepressant drugs for tissue and plasma proteins is that it is not possible to remove these agents by any known dialysis technique with sufficient speed to be of clinical benefit in the management of acute overdosage. By further analogy to the antipsychotic agents, the tricyclic antidepressants are metabolized mainly by oxidative mechanisms associated with hepatic microsomal enzyme systems. These reactions include ring hydroxylation and oxidation of the terminal amino nitrogen of the aliphatic side chain. Again, the general rule is that the oxidized products are more polar, more water soluble, and thus more readily excreted.

There have been attempts to utilize information about the pharmacokinetics and metabolism of the tricyclic antidepressants to improve their clinical effects. An important metabolic route is N-demethylation of imipramine and amitriptyline; the demethylated metabolites retain antidepressant activity and are available for clinical use as desmethyl- (or nor-) imipramine (Norpramin, Pertofrane) and desmethyl- (or nor-) amitriptyline (Aventyl) (Figure 5). Contrary to early hopes, neither agent is more rapid in onset than imipramine or amitriptyline; desmethylimipramine may not even be quite as effective as imipramine, and desmethylamitriptyline presents a moderate gain in potency (Table 10), but not efficacy. The demethylated antidepressants are somewhat less sedating, and this may reflect their greater selectivity and potency as inhibitors of norepinephrine intake.

Another application of pharmacokinetics has been the evaluation of blood levels of tricyclic antidepressants in an attempt to explain clinically disappointing results. There are clear, and presumably genetically determined, abilities to metabolize and excrete these agents; steady-state plasma concentrations vary between individuals by more than tenfold. There may be optimal blood levels of certain antidepressants (for example, 50–140 ng/ml of nortriptyline); either very low or very high levels may be correlated with diminished effectiveness. In Europe, these clinical correlations are considered sufficiently useful that blood levels of antidepressants are monitored almost routinely in some centers and interest is growing in the United States in the application of these methods, at least to patients who respond poorly to routine treatment with antidepressants.

A third application of basic pharmacology has been the attempt to alter the rate of metabolism of antidepressants with agents competing for hepatic microsomal enzymes. Phenothiazines and stimulants including methylphenidate (Ritalin) increase blood levels of tricyclic antidepressants, as do certain antibiotics and possibly even aspirin. In contrast, contraceptive hormones, other steroids, and barbiturates are capable of inducing increased amounts of several liver enzymes and decrease levels of antidepressants, presumably by increasing their hepatic metabolism. Although this work has been scientifically interesting, it has not yet led to convincing evidence that the clinical efficacy or safety of the tricyclic antidepressants can be altered by administering agents that interact with the hepatic microsomal enzymes. Moreover, the same ends might be achieved more simply by adjusting the dose of tricyclic drug.

The mechanisms of action of the antidepressant agents have been discussed. To recapitulate, the leading theory is that they block the uptake of amines acting in the brain as synaptic neurotransmitters or as local neurohormones, and thus the antidepressants potentiate the catecholamines and perhaps serotonin (5-hydroxytryptamine) while their muscarinic receptor blocking effects antagonize acetylcholine. The catecholamines are believed to have an important role in central mechanisms underlying sympathetic autonomic effects, drive states, appetitive behavior, arousal and the like, sometimes called "ergotropic" actions. Effects of the antidepressants on indoleamines including serotonin, and on acetylcholine may also contribute to antidepressant and other actions of the tricyclic drugs. The latter amines are centrally quieting, parasympathetic, or "trophotropic" neurohumors. Accordingly, the more sedating tricyclic antidepressants, including amitriptyline, chlorimipramine, and a number of other tricyclic methylated amines, have relatively great uptake-blocking and function-potentiating effects on serotonin, while the less sedating demethylated tricyclic agents such as desmethylimipramine and noramitriptyline exert preferential potentiating effects on norepinephrine.

The reason for the delay of several days to three weeks for the antidepressant clinical effects of these agents to appear is still uncertain. Furthermore, this delay presents a problem for the catecholamine hypothesis inasmuch as the catecholamine-potentiating actions of the drugs are immediate. The clinical delay might reflect the saturation of certain tissue pools, possibly at a crucial site on neuronal membranes.

Clinical Use

Treatment of depression is made difficult by the diversity of conditions subsumed under the generic term "depression," and by the inconsistency with which clinicians and investigators categorize depressions. Regardless of the scheme of categorization, it is generally agreed that depressions vary in severity. The more severe forms include those referred to as "endogenous," "manic-depressive," "retarded," "involutional," "agitated," "psychotic," or "vital," depending on the clinical form of the illness and the patient's history. In contrast, the less severe forms are said to be "minor," "reactive," "neurotic," "situational," or "anxious" depressions. Although the prognosis for the less severe depressions is better, efficacy of medical treatments has been more clearly demonstrated for the more serious depressions with more pronounced "biological" symptoms such as anorexia, insomnia, loss of drive and sexual interest, and diurnal change. The lesser depressive illnesses tend to recover more rapidly, to remit spontaneously and respond to psychotherapy, sedatives, antianxiety medications, stimulants, or to nonspecific treatments including placebos, about as well as to antidepressants. A difficulty in evaluating medical treatments of depression is that spontaneous remission rates for unselected depressions of various degrees of severity are about 20–25% within the first four to six weeks, and exceed 50% within a few months. Even severe depressions eventually underwent remission after many months in the era prior to ECT or antidepressant drugs. Moreover, adding a placebo increases remission rates of unselected acute depressions to about 40–50% in the first month or two.

The tricyclic antidepressants have their clearest effects in the more severe depressions, for which their performance in controlled clinical trials has been fairly consistent, although not dramatic (Table 11). The best performance of the drugs has been documented in trials that attempted to exclude the less severe depressions, used adequate doses of medication (more than 100 mg of imipramine or the equivalent of another agent), and continued for at least a month. In controlled trials with a

Table 10. Equivalent Doses of Tricyclic Antidepressants[a]

Generic Name	Trade Name	Dose Range (mg/day)
Amitriptyline	Elavil, etc., generic	50–300
Desipramine	Norpramin, Pertofrane	75–200
Doxepin	Adapin, Sinequan	75–300
Imipramine	Tofranil, etc., generic	50–300
Nortriptyline	Aventyl	50–100[b]
Protriptyline	Vivactil	15–60

a. Although the ratio of a severely toxic or lethal dose to a typical daily dose (approximate therapeutic index) may be as high as 10 to 30, 5 to 10 days' supply is a safer amount to dispense. Doses above 250 mg of amitriptyline, or the equivalent of other agents, are best reserved for inpatients. Daily doses are initially divided into two or three portions, but total doses of 150 mg or less can later be given at bedtime for convenience. Amitriptyline is available in combination with perphenazine (Etrafon, Triavil). Most commercial preparations are soluble hydrochlorides. Imipramine is also available as the slower acting pamoate (Tofranil-PM) that can be given in the same daily dose as the hydrochloride, in one or two portions, but it is more expensive and probably not safer than giving the hydrochloride twice a day or at bedtime. The usually effective dose is 150–200 mg of imipramine hydrochloride (or the equivalent of another agent) achieved over several days; smaller doses are used in children and elderly patients. In changing agents it is wise to make the conversion *gradually* over several days to avoid intoxication.

b. Recent studies suggest that optimal blood levels of nortriptyline are most commonly attained at a dose of 100–150 mg/day, although the manufacturer's current upper limit of recommended dosage is only 100 mg/day.

mixture of depressive syndromes of varying severity, overall improvement rates with tricyclic antidepressants have been about 70%, in contrast to about 40% with placebo: thus, only an additional 30% of patients with significant depressive illnesses respond to the active medication. A few who respond poorly to a tricyclic agent respond satisfactorily to an MAO inhibitor, and about half of those who respond poorly to a tricyclic agent respond to ECT. ECT has consistently outperformed MAO inhibitors or tricyclic antidepressants, but the overall gain is only on the order of 10–20%.

Among the specific antidepressants, there are more similarities than differences in overall effectiveness (Tables 11 and 12). The tricyclic antidepressants have performed better than MAO inhibitors, with the possible exception of tranylcypromine (Parnate), which has amphetamine-like properties as well as the ability to inhibit MAO and has produced results about equal to those of imipramine in a small number of comparisons (Table 11). Among the tricyclic antidepressants, amitriptyline (Elavil) may have produced somewhat better overall results than placebo in comparison with other tricyclic agents. Moreover, in direct comparisons of amitriptyline with imipramine, the former was somewhat more effective (Table 12). On the other hand, amitriptyline may be slightly slower in its onset than imipramine. Desmethylimipramine (Norpramin, Pertofrane) may be somewhat less effective than the other tricyclic agents. Thus, although desmethylimipramine was better than placebo in 66% of its controlled trials, imipramine was superior to its demethylated congener in 18% of 11 direct comparisons of the two agents (and about equal in the other 82%) (Table 12). There is no consistent evidence that the N-demethylated (nor-) derivatives of either imipramine or amitriptyline are more rapid in their onset than the parent compounds, but nortriptyline (Aventyl) may be slightly more potent (or toxic) than amitriptyline (Elavil) in that the recommended maximum dose is only 100 mg/day. Moreover, whereas another demethylated congener of amitriptyline, protriptyline (Vivactil), is more potent than either amitriptyline or nortriptyline, its overall efficacy is no greater than that of the other tricyclic antidepressants. Amitriptyline produces more sedation (at least initially) than most other antidepressants, and the demethylated antidepressants generally produce less, and may even have early stimulating actions; protriptyline may produce the least sedation. Amitriptyline has more potent anticholinergic activity than other tricyclic antidepressants, and desmethylimipramine (desipramine), the least, with other agents clustering between them. This consideration suggests that desipramine may be a more rational choice for elderly patients at high risk of anticholinergic brain syndrome, or of cardiac toxicity, although its greater safety has not been demonstrated clinically. The dibenzoxepine agent doxepin (Sinequan) has acquired an undeserved reputation for having special antianxiety or mixed antipsychotic and antidepressant qualities; much of this impression is based on its most successful use in outpatients with mild neurotic depressions and anxiety. This agent also has an unjustified reputation for not inhibiting uptake into noradrenergic neurons. Although *in vitro* studies support the generalization that the *di*methylated tricyclic antidepressants (imipramine and amitriptyline as well as doxepin) are less potent inhibitors of uptake into postganglionic sympathetic neurons than their demethylated or *mono*methylated analogues, these distinctions do not seem to make clinically important differences, perhaps because the *di*methylated compounds are readily converted *in vivo* to their *de*methylated metabolites. Specifically, the idea that doxepin does not block the uptake and hence the antihypertensive actions of the postganglionic sympathetic blocking agent guanethidine (Ismelin) is not correct, although this antihypertensive agent may be at least partially effective for the first two or three weeks of treatment with doxepin. The main conclusion based on these various comparisons is similar to that for the antipsychotic agents: although differences in the overall efficacy of the various tricyclic antidepressants are not easy to document, subtleties based on the relative chances for various side effects or drug interactions do call for some judgment and selecting a specific agent on the basis of sound pharmacological principles and clinical observations.

Recently it has been suggested that response to a specific antidepressant might possibly be predicted by a metabolic test. It had been suggested that an initial behavioral or cardiovascular

Table 11. Frequency with Which Treatments Proved More Effective
than Placebo for Depression

Agents	Percent of Trials Superior to Placebo[a]	Number of Controlled Trials
Tricyclics		
Imipramine	60	50
Desipramine	66	6
Amitriptyline	70	20
Nortriptyline	62	8
Protriptyline	100	3
Doxepin	100	1
Amitriptyline + perphenazine	80	5
MAO Inhibitors		
Tranylcypromine	75	4
Phenelzine	56	9
Other Treatments		
Amphetamines	0	3
Chlorpromazine	100	3
ECT	88	8

Source: Morris and Beck, *Arch. Gen. Psychiatry, 30* (1974), 667, © 1974,
American Medical Association; and Appleton and Davis, *Practical Clinical
Psychopharmacology,* Medcom Press, New York (© 1973), 106, with permis-
sion of The Williams & Wilkins Co.

a. Summarizes controlled studies of inpatients or outpatients with a variety
of depressive illnesses in which the agent produced results superior to a placebo statistically significant at least at $p \leq 0.05$.

activating response to amphetamine or other drugs might usefully predict response to a tricyclic antidepressant or to ECT,
although this approach has not been sufficiently powerful to
support its routine clinical application. More recently, an initially high excretion of MHPG, a urinary metabolite of norepinephrine (Figure 6), prior to treatment has been reported by

several researchers to correlate with a favorable response to amitriptyline, and lower levels of MHPG seem to predict a favorable response to imipramine. These differences in response do not simply correlate with "agitated" vs. "retarded" depressions contrary to what one might guess. Although the metabolic approach to predicting response to chemotherapy is potentially very important, biochemical tests such as MHPG excretion are still experimental techniques and are not yet applied routinely in clinical practice.

In selecting a specific agent for a specific case of depression, antipsychotic drugs must also be considered. In comparisons of tricyclic antidepressants and antipsychotic agents in groups of relatively unselected cases of serious depression, the overall benefits of the two types of agents have been about the same (Table 12). In one of the earliest studies, thioridazine was used, whereupon it acquired an exaggerated reputation as a specific agent for severe or psychotic depression. In fact, any antipsychotic agent will perform about as well as any antidepressant in such unselected comparisons, although comparisons of the same agents in schizophrenic patients yield poor results with the antidepressants. A trick in the comparison of antipsychotic and antidepressant agents is that the types of depressive syndromes specifically helped by the two classes of drugs are quite different. Antipsychotic agents are most helpful in cases of psychotic or involutional depression with a great deal of agitation and guilty or morbid rumination of delusional proportions. Tricyclic antidepressants are selectively useful for more quiet, ruminating, psychomotorically retarded depressions, as manic-depressive depressions usually are. Tricyclic antidepressants can even increase agitation in some cases of psychotic depression, and the addition or even exclusive use of an antipsychotic agent in the first few days or weeks of the treatment of such an illness can bring about more rapid benefits than a tricyclic antidepressant alone. The phenothiazine thioridazine (Mellaril) has also been reported to have beneficial effects in neurotic depressions, for which tricyclic antidepressants are sometimes helpful, but for which the benzodiazepines such as chlordiazepoxide or diazepam (Librium or Valium), are also useful and probably safer. It is not true that antidepresssant agents are so stimulating and behaviorally activating as to worsen the insomnia that typically accompanies serious depressions. Antidepressants even facilitate the deeper phases of sleep that are usually decreased in adult depression. On the other hand, imipramine in the management of childhood enuresis has been reported to be associated with a partial suppression of deeper phases of sleep. There is increased vulnerability of bipolar (or previously, apparently unipolar, sometimes called ''bipolar, type II'') manic-depressive patients to ''switch'' from retarded depression to mania in the course of treatment with a tricyclic antidepressant (or with stimulants or ECT). Conversely, the use of antipsychotic agents in mania (particularly haloperidol, probably as a reflection of its recent popularity for mania) has occasionally been complicated by the rapid switch from mania to depression; there is no reason to believe that any class of antipsychotic drugs is more likely to produce this effect, and it probably also occurs spontaneously in manic-depressive patients.

In schizophrenic illnesses, the place of antidepressant agents is not clearly defined. There has been a practice of trying at least moderate doses of antidepressants or L-dopa in withdrawn or apathetic schizophrenics, usually without clear benefits, and the antidepressants have been added to the treatment of more clearly depressive phases of schizophrenic or schizoaffective illnesses. These practices are not without risk, however, because stimulants, L-dopa, MAO inhibitors, and tricyclic antidepressants can increase or induce agitation, delusions, and hallucinations in schizophrenic and other psychotic

Table 12. Efficacy of Various Antidepressants Compared with Two Standard Agents[a]

	Imipramine			Amitriptyline		
Antidepressant	Percent Better[b]	Percent Similar[c]	N[d]	Percent Better[b]	Percent Similar[c]	N[d]
Imipramine	—	—	0	45	36	11
Desipramine	18	82	11	—	—	—
Amitriptyline	18	36	11	—	—	—
Nortriptyline	0	100	2	0	100	7
Protriptyline	0	100	2	33	67	6
Doxepin	0	100	3	12	50	8
Amitriptyline + perphenazine	0	0	1	17	67	6
Tranylcypromine	0	100	3	—	—	0
Phenelzine	56	44	9	—	—	0
ECT	0	57	7	—	—	0
Chlorpromazine	0	100	1	—	—	0
Thioridazine	0	100	1	—	—	0

Source: Morris and Beck, *Arch. Gen. Psychiatry, 30* (1976), 667, © 1976 American Medical Association; and Appleton and Davis, *Practical Clinical Psychopharmacology,* Medcom Press, New York (© 1973), 106, with permission of The Williams & Wilkins Co.

a. Summarizes controlled studies of inpatients and outpatients in which the agents were compared with imipramine or amitriptyline as standard antidepressants. ECT was consistently more effective than imipramine; most of the tricyclic agents produced similar results; amitriptyline may have a slight edge; the MAO inhibitor phenelzine seemed somewhat less effective than other agents at the doses used.

b. Percent of trials in which the *standard drug* gave *superior* results ($p \leq 0.05$).

c. Percent of trials in which two drugs gave similar results; results poorer than those of the standard agent account for the remaining variance (to total 100%) and are not tabulated.

d. N = number of *trials.*

patients, and occasionally antidepressants have been reported to be associated with the "uncovering of latent psychosis" in patients with schizoid, hysterical, paranoid, or "borderline" characters. Moreover, there is a risk of compounding a functional psychosis with an anticholinergic, toxic psychosis, particularly with daily doses of antidepressants above 200 mg of imipramine or the equivalent of another antidepressant, and with even lower doses if an antipsychotic agent and an anticholinergic antiparkinson agent are also being used.

The clinical use of antidepressant agents varies with the type of illness being treated. An elaborate medical evaluation before starting treatment is usually not helpful in younger and healthy individuals, but it is well to have a good appreciation of the cardiovascular, cerebrovascular, gastrointestinal, urinary, and ophthalmologic status of elderly depressed patients, who are at greater risk of toxic effects. Usually in outpatients or elderly patients, treatment is begun with moderate doses of the tricyclic agents. An initial daily dose as small as 25 mg/day of imipramine is extremely low, and 50–75 mg/day is typical. The amount is usually increased by 25 to 50 mg every day or two to doses of 100–150 mg/day of imipramine (or the equivalent of another agent; see Table 10). With inpatients it is more common to start with 100–150 mg and quickly reach doses of 150–250 mg/day. Doses above 200 or 250 mg/day of imipramine or its equivalent are associated with increased risks of toxic effects, including cardiovascular effects, psychotic agitation, and confusion, and are best reserved for carefully supervised, hospitalized patients, preferably after a trial of two or three weeks at 150–200 mg/day. In severe depression and when food and oral medications are refused, an injectable form of imipramine or amitriptyline can be used (initially, 100 mg/day in divided doses intramuscularly), although there is no compelling evidence that the efficacy or speed will be increased in that way. If there is psychosis or severe agitation, it is usually necessary to add an antipsychotic agent. There is little reason to add a hypnotic medication for sleep. If agitation and suicidal risk are high, several unilateral ECT's can be given while waiting for the effects of the antidepressant. Although ECT can be done safely while antidepressants are being used, it is wise to omit the first dose of antidepressant on the morning of ECT and use anticholinergic agents to dry secretions during ECT sparingly if at all. Although it might seem to be a good idea, it is not usual to give a stimulant in the first few days of hospitalization while awaiting the antidepressant effects of a tricyclic agent, because the benefits of amphetamine-like agents are meager, and there are added risks of inducing agitation and hypertension.

An important feature of *all antidepressant agents* is the *delay* in clinical onset of antidepressant effect, typically at least a week, sometimes up to three weeks. The failure of objective improvement in activity, sleep, appetite, mood, or social interest within a week is an unfavorable prognostic sign and suggests that the final result will be unsatisfactory. The patient is usually the last to acknowledge improvement, but if the objective response is poor after four or five weeks of adequate doses of a tricyclic agent, and if there is not even slight improvement in two or three weeks, there is little likelihood that changing to another agent or increasing doses above 300 mg of imipramine or its equivalent will help. At that point, the two main choices are to try an MAO inhibitor or ECT, and there is little reason not to go directly to ECT as it is more likely to have additional benefit. With outpatients, a period in a hospital at that point may also provide additional nonspecific benefits. If an MAO inhibitor is used, for example in a patient who refuses ECT, it is safer, but slower, to allow at least a week and, better, two weeks for the tricyclic agent to be metabolized and excreted before adding the MAO inhibitor to avoid the rare, but potentially catastrophic drug interactions, including hyperpyrexia and convulsions, that may occur.

The half-lives of the tricyclic agents are long enough that it is reasonable to use the bulk of a day's dose at bedtime, both for convenience and to combat insomnia. Furthermore, it is best to prescribe preparations of tricyclics with the highest unit strength (mg/pill) as this is usually the least expensive. For outpatients, the more slowly released pamoate salt of imipramine (Tofranil-PM) may also be used; its daily dose is the same as for the more usual soluble hydrochloride salt. This preparation is more expensive and does not offer a clear advantage over ordinary imipramine hydrochloride, which is available as a less expensive generic drug (Tofranil, Imavate, Presamine, SK-Pramine, and others). When large doses of an antidepressant are used (above the equivalent of 150 mg/day of imipramine), it is probably safer to use divided doses to minimize anticholinergic and cardiotoxic actions of the drugs, as well as nightmares, which occasionally follow large doses at bedtime. Similar to the antipsychotic agents, the clinically "equivalent doses" of antidepressant agents summarized in Table 10 have been established assuming that the doses are attained gradually. Thus, to avoid toxic reactions, it is best to avoid switching immediately from equivalent doses of one agent to another, and to allow several days for a gradual transition. Because of the potentially severe toxicity and limited margin of safety of all antidepressant agents, it is unwise to dispense more than a week's supply to a depressed and possibly suicidal outpatient. The risk of suicide may increase with initial improvement, since activity usually increases before mood elevation.

After appreciable clinical improvement of a severe depressive illness has been achieved with a tricyclic antidepressant agent, it is usual to *continue the treatment* at 100–150 mg/day of imipramine or its equivalent for several months, and perhaps up to a year for severe illness or in patients with a prior history of frequently recurrent depression. Doses as low as 75 mg in this phase of treatment are less effective in preventing relapses. A similar regimen should be followed by patients treated initially with ECT. This approach has evolved from clinical experience and many reports of relapse after partial treatment of depressions. The exact duration of the treatment depends on the individual patient's response, ability to resume normal responsibilities, premorbid personality, ongoing stresses and life situation, and the duration, rate of recurrence, and response to treatment of prior depressions. There is encouraging evidence that the sustained use of tricyclic agents in unipolar manic-depressive illness (Table 13) may be as useful as lithium is in preventing or diminishing bipolar or unipolar illnesses (Table 7), although the efficacy and safety of indefinitely prolonged antidepressant therapy are not fully established. The usefulness of indefinitely continued treatment in outpatients with "chronic characterological depressions" is not clear, although this is occasionally done.

Attempts have been made to increase the efficacy or the rapidity of onset of antidepressant agents. Thyroid status may alter the efficacy of antidepressants, and thyroid function

Table 13. Rate of Relapse of Unipolar Depression with Tricyclic Antidepressants or Placebo

Treatment	N^a	Relapsed	Percent Relapsed	Mean Relapse Rate ± SEM (Percent)
Antidepressant[b]	162	44	27.2	28.1 ± 8.9[c]
Placebo	202	107	53.0	59.7 + 9.4

Source: J. M. Davis, Am. J. Psychiatry, 133 (1976), 1.

a. N = number of patients in controlled studies, a total of 364 patients.

b. Tricyclic antidepressants included imipramine or amitriptyline. Placebo included inert tablet or diazepam.

c. $p < 2 \times 10^{-8}$, comparing results for antidepressant vs. placebo, using pooled data.

should be evaluated in patients who fail to respond to adequate doses of an antidepressant within about a month. The addition of thyroid hormone, for example, 25 μg of *l*-triiodothyronine (Cytomel), even to euthyroid patients might improve the response to tricyclic antidepressants in some *female* patients, although this approach increases the risk of cardiac toxicity in patients at high risk, such as the elderly or those with prior myocardial infarction. Thyroid-stimulating hormone (TSH) may have a similar effect, and hypothalamic thyrotropin-releasing factor (TRF) may itself have mood elevating and even antidepressant effects when given intravenously, although these effects have not been replicated consistently. For the present, while the search continues for more effective and safer antidepressant therapies, the cornerstones of the medical therapy of severe depressive illness are the tricyclic antidepressants and ECT.

Tricyclic antidepressants have also been used for conditions other than depression. The usefulness of MAO inhibitors and tricyclic agents in certain phobic neuroses has been reported. These agents and ECT are occasionally helpful in some pain syndromes that might represent "depressive equivalents," as well as in migraine, narcolepsy, and in other psychosomatic conditions. Several disorders of children including enuresis, school phobias, and a variety of "nervous habits" have been treated with antidepressants, especially with doses of imipramine of 25–75 mg/day, an hour or more before bedtime.

Depression is very common, but frequently overlooked in elderly patients who can be treated with tricyclic antidepressants or, in cases marked by agitation, with antipsychotic agents. In the elderly, depression can present signs and symptoms that mimic dementia, and it may occur in addition to underlying senile changes. It is important to respond to reversible and treatable forms of mood change in senescence, so as to avoid secondary complications including malnutrition, withdrawal, and isolation. Somatic and hypochondriacal symptoms are common and occur early. Improvement in behavior and cognition, and decreased hypochondriasis are useful indicators of a therapeutic response to antidepressants in the elderly. Stimulants such as amphetamine and methylphenidate have no place in treating the elderly, and usually produce a worsening of affect, dysphoria, agitation, confusion, anorexia, and paranoia. The tricyclic antidepressants frequently produce serious side effects in the elderly, particularly organic mental syndromes and anticholinergic effects, and so are used in smaller, and gradually increased, divided doses. Amitriptyline and thioridazine have been popular medications for the treatment of depressive syndromes in the elderly, but should be avoided due to their strong anticholinergic actions. Doxepin has recently been advocated as a relatively safe antidepressant for elderly patients, and desmethylimipramine may be relatively safe due to its weak anticholinergic activity. When agitation and paranoia are prominent signs, a high-potency antipsychotic agent (to avoid the excessive sedation and hypotension of less potent drugs) may be preferable, because of the tendency for tricyclic antidepressants to provoke agitation, increase paranoia, or induce delirium.

In children, the tricyclic antidepressants have not been well evaluated except for the treatment of enuresis and hyperactivity. It is particularly difficult to define specific target symptoms of depression in children, and even the existence of depression in children that is analogous to the adult syndromes is debated. Antidepressants have been claimed to modify a wide variety of misbehavior in children, some forms of which may represent depressive illnesses, although this concept and form of treatment are not well established. In some autistic, psychotic, or brain-damaged children, antidepressants have a deleterious, mentally disorganizing action. Antidepressants are being evaluated as an experimental treatment of anorexia nervosa in adolescents.

Side Effects and Toxicity

Important toxic effects occur in perhaps 5% of patients treated with tricyclic antidepressants; of these, more than 10% represent cerebral intoxication, and the incidence of nervous system toxicity is much higher over the age of forty. The most common toxic side effects of the tricyclic antidepressants are extensions of their pharmacologic activities. These include anticholinergic actions leading to dry mouth, sweating, and ophthalmologic changes. The latter are variable but usually include mild mydriasis and often some degree of cycloplegia with blurred near vision because of impaired accommodation. These problems are more annoying than dangerous and can usually be managed by simple means such as candy or mild mouth washes to offset reduced salivation, and reading lenses to compensate for reduced near vision. Cholinergic eye drops, cholinergic mouth washes, or systemic medications have been tried for these various symptoms, but are usually not very helpful. Moreover, some degree of tolerance to the side effects normally develops. The overuse of candy for dry mouth can lead to monilial infections. Grossly excessive water intake secondary to dry mouth on rare occasions can lead to water intoxication due to significant hyponatremia, particularly in confused patients. Water intoxication also occurs infrequently with the use of antipsychotic drugs; it is not yet clear whether this effect is due to endocrinologic effects of antidepressant or antipsychotic agents, such as an inappropriate increase in the release of antidiuretic hormone (ADH).

Among more serious aspects of the anticholinergic actions of antidepressants is the induction of *glaucoma,* as with the antipsychotic agents. *Serious antivagal effects* of this highly anticholinergic class of agents include paralytic ileus and urinary retention; thus extra caution is required in elderly patients and men with prostatism, and urgent medical intervention is necessary when these conditions develop. Treatment entails eliminating or reducing the dose of antidepressant, giving cholinergic smooth-muscle stimulants such as bethanechol (Urecholine), 2.5 or 5.0 mg subcutaneously as needed. When severe inhibition of gastrointestinal or urinary function occurs with even small doses of antidepressants, it may be necessary to change the treatment to ECT or an MAO inhibitor. Among the tricyclic agents, desipramine has the least peripheral and CNS antimuscarinic activity in animal tissues, while amitriptyline is the most potently anticholinergic: about 5% the potency of atropine, but given in doses more than 100 times greater than atropine (Table 14). It is not yet certain whether these differences are significant clinically, however.

Various *skin* reactions have been described, and an allergic-obstructive type of *jaundice* occasionally occurs early in the course of treatment. Purpura has been reported in a few cases. *Agranulocytosis* is rare. There may be a tendency to gain weight, and there are occasional hypoglycemic effects of the tricyclic agents.

A serious consequence of the anticholinergic and direct quinidine-like properties of the tricyclic antidepressants is their *cardiac toxicity*. Palpitations, tachycardia and arrhythmias are not unusual and are to be expected in cases of acute overdosage. EKG changes include tachycardia, prolongation of the Q-T interval and flattening of the T waves. The myocardium is often directly depressed; decreased strength of contraction creates some risk of syncope. Faintness due to postural hypotension also is not unusual, although the underlying mechanisms are not clear. Steroids such as cortisone, as well as dihydroergotamine (10 mg/day), have been reported to counteract postural hypotension resulting from administration of tricyclic antidepressants or MAO inhibitors when more conservative management did not suffice. Because there is an increased risk of malignant ventricular arrhythmias, cardiac arrest, left ventricular enlargement, myocardial dam-

Table 14. Antimuscarinic Potency of
CNS Agents[a]

Agent	EC_{50} (nM)[b]
Scopolamine	0.3
Atropine	0.4
Trihexyphenidyl (Artane)	0.6
Benztropine (Cogentin)	1.5
Amitriptyline (Elavil)	10
Doxepin (Sinequan)	44
Nortriptyline (Aventyl)	57
Imipramine (Tofranil)	78
Desipramine (Norpramin)	170
Clozapine	26
Thioridazine (Mellaril)	150
Promazine (Sparine)	650
Chlorpromazine (Thorazine)	1000
Triflupromazine (Vesprin)	1000
Acetophenazine (Tindal)	10,000
Perphenazine (Trilafon)	11,000
Fluphenazine (Prolixin)	12,000
Trifluoperazine (Stelazine)	13,000
Haloperidol (Haldol)	48,000
Iproniazid (Marplan)	>100,000
Nialamid (Niamid)	>100,000
Phenelzine (Nardil)	>100,000

Source: S. Snyder, D. Greenberg, and H. Yamamura, *Arch. Gen. Psychiatry, 31* (1974), 58; and *34* (1977), 236, © 1974 and 1977, American Medical Association.

a. Estimated in rat brain homogenates by assay of competition with the binding of the avid and selective muscarinic antagonist [³H]-3-quinuclidinylbenzilate (QNB).

b. Data are half-maximally effective concentrations (EC_{50}) of drugs which compete for the binding to tissue of the labeled test agent, ³H-QNB. Conconcentrations are in units of nM (nanomolar, or $10^{-9}M$).

age, and congestive heart failure with the tricyclic antidepressants, they must be used in lower doses and with great caution in elderly patients at risk for myocardial infarction and stroke, and avoided after myocardial infarction. Amitriptyline may be particularly cardiotoxic, although this impression derives from studies in animals. An important consideration in choosing the treatment for serious depression in elderly or infirm patients is that with its modern modifications, ECT is probably as safe as the antidepressant drugs if not safer. Mortality rates with the tricyclic agents and ECT are both low, but the incidence of serious morbidity and mortality with the drugs may even be higher than with ECT if overdoses are included; certainly the total morbidity rate with the drugs is considerable, especially if minor as well as more serious toxic effect and overdosages are all taken into account.

The untoward effects of tricyclic antidepressants on the *central nervous system* include mild dizziness and lightheadedness, insomnia and restlessness, or fatigue and somnolence. Fine and occasionally gross resting tremors are common and may respond to diazepam (Valium), but extrapyramidal syndromes are rare, possibly as a reflection of the powerful anticholinergic action of these drugs. The latter action is sufficient to produce antiparkinson effects, which are occasionally encountered when antidepressants are combined with neuroleptic agents or when they are given to depressed patients with Parkinson's disease. Tricyclic antidepressants must be used with caution by patients receiving antiparkinson medications due to the risk of combined anticholinergic toxicity. They would be expected to worsen choreas, including tardive dyskinesia, as antiparkinson drugs often do. There is some risk of provoking or worsening agitation and psychosis in patients with psychotic or unstable characterological conditions in addition to depression, and large doses or acute overdoses of the tricyclic antidepressants can induce a toxic organic psychosis resembling that due to atropine poisoning (Table 15). This toxic state is not always easy to diagnose in severely depressed patients who are already agitated and psychotic. Seizures and the worsening of epilepsy have also been associated with the antidepressants. Large doses of tricyclics at bedtime may produce nightmares. Withdrawal reactions have been reported to follow the abrupt discontinuation of high doses of tricyclic antidepressants (rare unless doses exceed 300 mg/day of imipramine or its equivalent); they include restlessness, anxiety, and akathisia but almost never seizures. Thus it is best to discontinue unusually high doses *slowly*.

The agents used in the treatment of mood disorders (tricyclic antidepressants, MAO inhibitors, and lithium salts) are much more toxic in *acute overdosage* than the antipsychotic agents, and unfortunately, must be given to patients at increased risk of attempting suicide. The tricyclic antidepressants are an increasingly common choice in suicide attempts by increasingly younger persons. Acute doses above 1000 mg are almost always very toxic, but doses as low as a few hundred mg, especially of amitriptyline, have been severely toxic in adults as well as children. Acute doses in excess of 2000 mg can be fatal. The monomethylated (*de*methylated) derivatives may be slightly less toxic than the *di*methylated parent compounds. Because of the relatively low therapeutic index, or margin of safety, of all tricyclic antidepressants, it is unwise to dispense more than a week's supply, and certainly never more than 1000 mg of imipramine or the equivalent of another agent (Table 10).

After an acute overdose, it is impossible to remove these agents by dialysis; forced diuresis adds little and may contribute to cardiac failure. Although attempts to increase the dialysis of antidepressants by the use of oils, resins, or charcoal have not been successful, activated charcoal is sometimes introduced into the gut during gastric lavage in an attempt to bind and inactivate any remaining unabsorbed drugs.

Severe central nervous system depression and coma (rarely lasting more than twenty-four hours) can result from large doses of the antidepressants, but it is common to see signs of *anticholinergic poisoning* early, with restless agitation, confusion, disorientation, perhaps seizures and hyperthermia, dry, sometimes flushed skin, tachycardia, sluggish and at least moderately dilated pupils, decreased bowel sounds, and often acute urinary retention (Table 15). These effects are probably due to CNS and systemic anticholinergic and antivagal actions of these potent muscarinic blocking agents. The *cardiac toxicity* can be particularly dangerous, and includes severe depression of myocardial conduction, with various forms of heart block, atrial fibrillation and more malignant ventricular arrhythmias or cardiac arrest. A peculiarity of tricyclic poisoning is that the risk of cardiac arrhythmias continues at least several days, and possibly up to a week or more after the initial brain syndrome has cleared considerably. Many of the agents commonly employed to manage ventricular arrhythmias can lead to further conduction blockade and cardiac depression. Electrical defibrillation, conversion and cardiac pacing may be necessary, and all cases of moderate to severe tricyclic poisoning should ideally be managed in a medical intensive care unit, with constant cardiac monitoring, excellent medical and cardiological supervision, and immediately available defibrillating and resuscitation equipment. It is also wise to continue cardiac monitoring for several days after the initial recovery of consciousness and orientation, perhaps up to seven to ten days in severe cases. Whereas many cardiac drugs, including digitalis, are contraindicated or dangerous, both the cardiac and central nervous system manifestations of anticholinergic poisoning can be successfully treated with reversible anticholinesterase agents. Neostigmine (Prostigmin) and pyridostigmine (Mestinon) have been successfully used in the management of the cardiac effects of a number of atropine-like agents, including

Table 15. Anticholinergic and Cholinergic Excess Syndromes

Anticholinergic Syndrome

Causes

Acute overdose or excessive prescription of medications with antimuscarinic properties, especially in combination: tricyclic antidepressants, most antiparkinson agents, some antipsychotics (especially thioridazine), many proprietary sedative-hypnotics, many antispasmodic preparations, several plants (e.g., Jimson weed, some mushrooms).

Neuropsychiatric Signs

Anxiety, agitation; restless, purposeless overactivity; delirium, disorientation; impairment of immediate and recent memory; dysarthria; hallucinations; myoclonus; seizures.

Systemic Signs

Tachycardia and arrhythmias, large sluggish pupils, scleral injection, flushed warm dry skin, increased temperature, decreased mucosal secretions; urinary retention, reduced bowel motility.

Treatment

Adults: initial or test dose: 1–2 mg physostigmine salicylate, intramuscularly, or *slowly* intravenously; repeat as needed after at least 15–30 minutes.

Children: 0.5–1.0 mg physostigmine salicylate, as for adults. (Neostigmine, pyridostigmine, etc., do not enter the CNS.)

Physostigmine-Induced Cholinergic Excess

Neuropsychiatric Signs

Confusion, seizures, nausea and vomiting, myoclonus, hallucinations, often after a period of initial CNS improvement when physostigmine is given to treat the anticholinergic syndrome.

Systemic Signs

Bradycardia, miosis, increased mucosal secretions, copious bronchial secretions, dyspnea, tears, sweating, diarrhea, abdominal colic, biliary colic, urinary frequency or urgency.

Treatment or Prevention

Atropine sulfate (CNS + systemic actions): 0.5 mg per mg of physostigmine, intramuscularly or subcutaneously.

Methscopolamine bromide (Pamine) (no CNS action): 0.5 mg per mg of physostigmine, intramuscularly.

Glycopyrrolate (Robinul) (no CNS action): 0.1 to 0.2 mg per mg of physostigmine, intramuscularly.

tricyclic antidepressants and antiparkinson agents. However, these anticholinesterase drugs are charged quaternary ammonium compounds that poorly penetrate the blood-brain barrier, and *only physostigmine* (eserine, Antilirium) has both central and peripheral cholinergic activity. Physostigmine therefore represents the treatment of choice in the management of intoxications with agents possessing significant anticholinergic activity. The principles of its use are outlined in Table 15. There is a recent report that prolonged coma due to an antidepressant, without prominent anticholinergic signs, was helped by large doses of physostigmine.

Other aspects of the pharmacology of the tricyclics should also be appreciated in the management of their overdoses. For example, the ability of these compounds to potentiate directly sympathomimetic amines such as norepinephrine complicates the use of such pressor substances in managing the hypotension and shock of tricyclic poisoning. Furthermore, the tricyclic agents potentiate and prolong the actions of barbiturates, probably through competition for hepatic microsomal enzymes, which are particularly important in inactivating the shorter-acting barbiturates. Although small doses of very short-acting barbiturates have been advocated for the control of seizures associated with tricyclic poisoning, diazepam (Valium) is probably a safer anticonvulsant in this situation and is less likely to induce respiratory depression.

Tricyclic agents have many *interactions with other drugs* (Table 16). Tricyclic antidepressants increase the CNS depression caused by alcohol, barbiturates, and some minor tranquilizers as well as antipsychotic agents and anticonvulsants. The barbiturates and glutethimide (Doriden) much more than the benzodiazepines also induce hepatic microsomal enzymes required for the metabolism of the tricyclic agents, and thus may decrease the efficacy of the tricyclics. The seizure threshold may be lowered, so increased doses of anticonvulsants may be

Table 16. Interactions[a] of Psychopharmaceuticals with Other Agents

Agent	Neuroleptic Antipsychotics	Tricyclic Antidepressants	MAO Inhibitors
Alcohol, anxiolytics, antihistamines	More sedation	More sedation and anticholinergic effects	More sedation, decreased metabolism
Anesthetics	Potentiate hypotension	Cardiac arrhythmias (?)	Potentiate
Barbiturates	More sedation, increase metabolism of neuroleptic	More sedation and anticholinergic, increase metabolism of antidepressant	More sedation, decrease metabolism of MAO inhibitors
Narcotics, especially meperidine	Potentiate	Some potentiation	Dangerous CNS depression or excitation and fever
Anticonvulsants	Make less effective	Make less effective	CNS depression
Anticholinergics, antiparkinson agents, spasmolytics	Unpredictable, decreased absorption of neuroleptics?	Potentiate each other, more anticholinergic effects	Potentiate, CNS intoxication; decrease metabolism of MAO inhibitors
L-dopa	Antagonize each other	Decrease absorption	May induce hypertension
Stimulants, anorexics	Antagonize each other, decrease metabolism of neuroleptics	Potentiate, induce hypertension, decrease metabolism of tricyclics	CNS excitation, hypertension, fever
Reserpine	Some potentiation of each other	Acutely, hypertension; later some inhibition; arrhythmias (?)	Paradoxical hypertension and CNS excitation acutely

(continued on next page)

Table 16. (continued)

Agent	Neuroleptic Antipsychotics	Tricyclic Antidepressants	MAO Inhibitors
Alpha-methyldopa	Potentiate each other	May antagonize	Paradoxical hypertension
Alpha-methyltyrosine	May potentiate antipsychotics; sedation	—	—
Guanethidine, bethanidine, debrisoquine	Some antagonism and withdrawal hypotension	Antagonize, severe withdrawal hypotension	Potentiate; acute hypertension with guanethidine
Hypotensive diuretics	More hypotension	—	More hypotension
Hypotensive smooth muscle relaxants (e.g., hydralazine)	More hypotension		More hypotension
Any agent with *MAO inhibitory* action (e.g., Eutonyl, Furoxone, Matulane)	Potentiate, hypo- or hypertension, extrapyramidal symptoms	Seizures, hyperpyrexia	Additive toxicity
Alpha-adrenergic agonists (e.g., norepinephrine, phenylephrine)	Make less effective	Potentiate	Potentiate
Clonidine (Catapres)	Potentiate (?)	Antagonize (mechanism unknown)	Potentiate (?)
Indirect sympathomimes (e.g., tyramine in food)	Some antagonism	Antagonize	Hypertension, CNS excitation, stroke
Alpha-adrenergic blockers (e.g., phentolamine, phenoxybenzamine)	Potentiate, hypotension	Antagonize	Antagonize

Agent			Potentiate[b]
Beta-adrenergic agonists (e.g., epinephrine, isoproterenol)	Hypotension	Potentiate	Antagonize acutely, potentiate later
Beta-adrenergic blockers (e.g., propranolol)	Hypotension	Antagonize	Probably potentiate
Anticoagulants (e.g., coumarins and indanediones)	Potentiate, decrease metabolism (withdrawal bleeding)	Minimal potentiation	?
Cardiac agents (e.g., quinidine, digitalis)	May potentiate	May potentiate	?
Steroids	—	Unpredictable	?
Insulin and *oral hypoglycemics*	Potentiate or inhibit	Unpredictable, may potentiate	Potentiate
Oral alkalis (e.g., Amphojel) and *resins* (e.g., Cholestyramine, Questran)	Absorption of neuroleptics decreased	Absorption of tricyclics decreased	?

a. Unless otherwise stated, effects are those of the psychopharmaceutical on actions of the medical agents in the first column. Dash indicates no effect known; question mark indicates no effects clearly demonstrated, but should be suspected.

b. Beware of administering dental preparations of procaine (Novocain) containing epinephrine (adrenaline) to patients receiving MAO inhibitors.

required. The effect of any anticholinergic agent (including antiparkinson drugs) will be additively increased by the antimuscarinic activity of the tricyclic antidepressants, and this combination creates a risk of toxic confusional brain syndrome, agitation, and sometimes hyperpyrexia. Antipsychotic agents are contraindicated in cases of toxic agitation produced by overdoses of tricyclic antidepressants due to their own moderate anticholinergic actions.

A difficult combination to manage satisfactorily is *depression and hypertension.* Antihypertensive agents possibly because of their central antiadrenergic properties, are sometimes associated with depression. This association may occur unpredictably at any point in the treatment of hypertension; it is most common in patients with a prior history of depression. It has most frequently been reported with reserpine and other *Rauwolfia* alkaloids, and occasionally with alpha-methyldopa (Aldomet). Guanethidine is one of the few antihypertensive agents with little CNS activity and is not likely to induce or worsen depression, although, surprisingly, sporadic anecdotal reports of its association with depression exist. Owing to blockade by tricyclics of guanethidine uptake into postganglionic sympathetic nerve fibers (Table 16), the treatment of hypertension with guanethidine in patients who are also depressed is usually rendered unsuccessful by the addition of any of the currently available tricyclic antidepressants (and to some extent the phenothiazines as well, but less so haloperidol or molindone). Although doxepin (Sinequan) has been claimed to have this effect much less than the other antidepressants, the claim is at best only partially valid for small doses of the antidepressant (less than 150 mg/day) for brief periods of time (less than two or three weeks). The antihypertensive effects of a number of other agents, including reserpine and the veratrum alkaloids, can also be diminished by the tricyclic antidepressants. It is safe to use diuretics with tricyclic antidepressants for the management of hypertension in depressed patients, although there is at least one report that moderate degrees of hyponatremia have depressant effects. It is also possible to treat hypertension with large doses of a beta-adrenergic blocking agent such as propranolol (Inderal) combined with the vascular smooth-muscle relaxant hydralazine (Apresoline); but high doses of the former can produce central sedative effects and may induce depression, and hydralazine has occasionally induced toxic psychoses. However, this combination of antihypertensive agents with tricyclic antidepressants has not yet been evaluated. One other approach to the management of depression with hypertension might be to take advantage of the hypotensive effects of MAO inhibitors, and particularly the nonhydrazine, pargyline (Eutonyl), which was initially withdrawn as an antidepressant because of its hypotensive effects and later relicensed as an antihypertensive agent. However, this use of pargyline has not yet been adequately evaluated; moreover, it must be used *alone* to avoid the risk of such potentially severe toxic interactions of an MAO inhibitor with a tricyclic antidepressant as hypertension, seizures, and hyperthermia.

The safety of antidepressant drugs in *pregnancy and lactation* is not established. They pass the placental barrier and can be secreted at low levels in human milk. In severe pre- and postpartum depression, ECT can safely be used. There have been rare reports of neonatal distress in infants born to mothers given antidepressants; these reactions included muscle spasms, myoclonus, tachycardia, congestive heart failure, and respiratory distress.

Because of their decreased ability to metabolize drugs of all types, and probably as an expression of decreased functional "resilience" of the central nervous system, elderly patients treated with tricyclic antidepressants are particularly likely to experience toxic side effects. Delirium and agitation are common, partly as an expression of the central anticholinergic syndrome, which should be suspected if there are signs of peripheral vagal and ciliary blockade and evaluated pharmacologically with a small test dose of physostigmine (Table 15). If this syndrome develops, antipsychotic agents are avoided, and management is either conservative (to allow time for elimination of the offending agent), or treatment is begun with small doses of physostigmine, or in uncertain cases with diazepam. Hypotension, cardiac arrhythmias, and glaucoma are also particularly likely in elderly patients. One other commonly encountered situation is the simultaneous use of anticoagulants with tricyclic agents, which may interfere with hepatic metabolism of the anticoagulants and thus increase their activity and the risk of bleeding (Table 16), although recent studies have concluded that this effect is minor and unlikely to be clinically important.

MAO Inhibitors and CNS Stimulants

Inhibitors of the enzyme *monoamine oxidase* (MAO) (Figure 7, Table 17) are historically important as they had a major impact on the medical treatment of depression and on the biological theories that attempt to relate brain metabolism to psychiatric illness. In 1952 the first useful antidepressant, iproniazid (Marsilid), was introduced in Europe and its inhibitory effects on MAO were described. A few years later, the ability of reserpine to deplete serotonin and norepinephrine in the mammalian brain while inducing behavioral "depression" was noted by B. B. Brodie and P. A. Shore at the U. S. National Institutes of Health; speculation then began that a functional deficiency of brain amines may underlie depression and that MAO inhibitors and other antidepressants act by reversing this deficiency. This view was formulated very early by N. Kline, who, simultaneously with several other American investigators, demonstrated the usefulness of iproniazid in serious depression. Since that time, the MAO inhibitors have fallen into a position of very limited use. The tricyclic agents are consistently superior as antidepressants (Table 11) and do not have the serious toxic effects of the MAO inhibitors. Several MAO inhibitors, including iproniazid, have been removed from the market because of severe hepatocellular toxicity, limited efficacy, or hypotensive effects. Moreover, these agents are severely toxic on acute overdosage and can induce dangerous interactions with other drugs, chemicals, hormones, or metabolic conditions (Table 16). Although the likelihood of inducing serious drug reactions with an MAO inhibitor is small (the overall fatality rate is about 0.001%), and even lower than serious morbidity due to ECT or the tricyclic antidepressants, the reactions are serious and potentially fatal when they do occur. Thus the dangers of toxicity, the inconvenience of restrictions required for the safe use of MAO inhibitors, and the limited efficacy of these agents in serious depression have resulted in their near abandonment in this country.

In controlled trials of the currently available MAO inhibitors, their efficacy has been consistently inferior to that of ECT and the tricyclic antidepressants. They produced results significantly better than a placebo in only 38% of the published trials overall, although these results for individual agents ranged from no superiority over a placebo for nialamide to superior results in 75% of trials of tranylcypromine (Table 11). Moreover, imipramine proved to be superior in 40% to 100% of comparisons with specific MAO inhibitors other than tranylcypromine (Table 12). An exception to these rather dismal results has been the amphetamine-like nonhydrazine MAO inhibitor, tranylcypromine (Parnate), which has outperformed a placebo in three of four studies and was found equal to imipramine in antidepressant efficacy in three of three studies. Whereas most antidepressants and MAO inhibitors require one to three weeks to produce beneficial effects, tranylcypromine usually acts within a few days, possibly because of its amphetamine-like stimulant actions. The only other MAO inhibitor presently in common use as an antidepressant in this country, in addition to tranylcypromine, is phenelzine (Nardil). In recent trials, when given at doses above 50 mg/day, it has performed almost as well as the tricyclics as an antidepressant. In contrast to the MAO inhibitors, most tricyclic antidepressants have produced better results than a placebo in nearly 80% of their 93 controlled clinical trials, and ECT has been effective nearly 90% of its controlled trials.

At present, the main indication for the use of MAO inhibitors is as a second choice of medication when a vigorous trial of a tricyclic antidepressant has been unsatisfactory. This step requires a *delay of at least 7–10 days after stopping the tricyclic* agent to permit its metabolism and excretion to avoid the rare but potentially severe interactions with MAO inhibitors.

HYDRAZINE

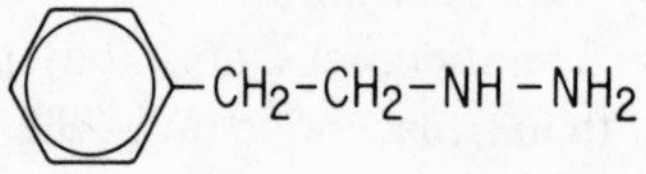

$$\bigcirc\!\!-CH_2-CH_2-NH-NH_2$$

Phenelzine (Nardil)

NON-HYDRAZINE

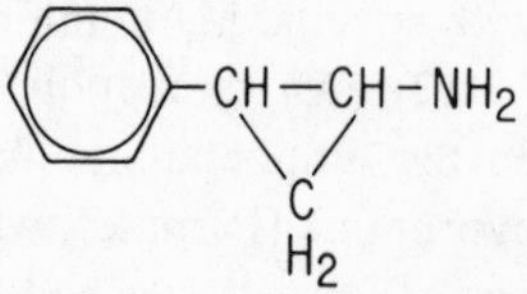

$$\bigcirc\!\!-CH-CH-NH_2$$
$$\underset{H_2}{C}$$

Tranylcypromine (Parnate)

Figure 7. Monoamine oxidase inhibitors

The MAO inhibitors are rapidly metabolized and excreted; however, because the hydrazine MAO inhibitors such as phenelzine are irreversible enzyme inhibitors and it takes a week or more to resynthesize new active molecules of MAO, a delay of 2 weeks is safer before giving a tricyclic antidepressant after an MAO inhibitor. Pargyline (Eutonyl), a nonhydrazine hypotensive agent, is also an irreversible MAO inhibitor with a prolonged action. Recovery of MAO activity after tranylcypromine, a nonhydrazine, is as rapid as two or three days.

As as general rule, it is better to hospitalize patients and to add ECT for cases of serious depressions responding poorly after several weeks of an adequate dose of a tricyclic agent. If an MAO inhibitor is to be used, at present tranylcypromine is the most effective antidepressant, the most rapid in onset of its clinical effects and termination of its chemical effect. It is also about the most toxic on acute overdosage. An additional reason to consider tranylcypromine as an initial therapy for severe depression is that it lacks the severe anticholinergic and potentially cardiotoxic effects of the tricyclic agents; thus it offers a *theoretical* advantage in elderly patients with heart disease, provided that contact with sympathomimetic agents can be scrupulously avoided, and provided that hypotension does not complicate the treatment. Phenelzine (Nardil) is a reasonable alternative if it is used in doses of 50 to 75 mg/day.

Some psychiatrists have claimed special effects of the MAO inhibitors in certain states, conditions that are not necessarily depressions and are marked by neurotic *anxiety and phobia* in adults or children, although tricyclic antidepressants may produce similar results. This use of MAO inhibitors in adults is particularly well thought of in England, where MAO inhibitors and tricyclic antidepressants are also sometimes combined. Nevertheless, the combination of MAO inhibitors or stimulants with tricyclic antidepressants cannot be recommended as a safe practice unless further experimental data become available to support the safety and additional benefits of this approach.

When MAO inhibitors are used clinically, both minor and serious *toxic effects* may be encountered. Hypotensive effects, usually *orthostatic hypotension* are usually a relatively minor problem. They may result from gradual accumulation in sympathetic nerve endings of amines lacking direct sympathomimetic activity at the expense of the normal synaptic transmitter, norepinephrine (this is a "false transmitter" hypothesis). The hypotensive effects of MAO inhibitors can usefully be applied

Table 17. MAO Inhibitors and Stimulants; Equivalent Dosage, and Approximate Therapeutic Index

Generic Name	Trade Name	Dose Range (mg/day)	Ratio of Lethal to Daily Dose[a]
MAO Inhibitors [b]			
Isocarboxazid	Marplan[c]	10–30	10–15
Phenelzine	Nardil[c]	15–75	5–10
Tranylcypromine	Parnate[d]	10–30	6
Stimulants			
d-Amphetamine	Dexedrine, etc. (generic)	10–20	10–50
Methylphenidate	Ritalin	20–30	10–50

a. The ratio of lethal to daily doses (approximate therapeutic index) is an estimate, based on reports of severe intoxication and lethality in adults, and suggests the number of days' supply that may be dispensed safely; ratios for children are two to five times *lower*.

b. Other MAO inhibitors have been used but are no longer marketed (Catron, Marsilid, Monase, Niamid), or are not used in psychiatry (Eutonyl, Eutron, Furoxone, Matulane).

c. The effectiveness of the recommended doses of Marplan or of low doses of Nardil (<45 mg/day) compared to placebo is not certain.

d. Not recommended over age 60 or in cardiac patients.

to the treatment of moderate forms of hypertension and this has been done with pargyline (Eutonyl). On the other hand, the hypotension may become worrisome in patients at high risk of heart attack or stroke. The diminution of sympathetically regulated arteriolar tone may also contribute to the reported antianginal effects of most MAO inhibitors. Severe *parenchymal hepatotoxic* reactions occur infrequently and are generally much more serious than the biliary stasis associated with antipsychotic and tricyclic antidepressant agents. This toxicity is serious enough to justify frequent, perhaps weekly, determinations of serum bilirubin and transaminase activities, and to contraindicate the use of MAO inhibitors in patients with chronic liver disease to whom small doses of tricyclic antidepressants can be cautiously given. Manifestations of *CNS toxicity* include agitation, insomnia, and toxic psychoses, as well as provocation of previously quiescent functional psychoses.

The most serious toxic effect of the MAO inhibitors (particularly tranylcypromine) is their ability to provoke *acute hypertensive crises,* sometimes with hyperpyrexia, seizures, intracranial bleeding, and cardiovascular collapse. These catastrophic reactions are fortunately rare, and can largely be prevented by scrupulous avoidance of *medications, foods, and beverages* with appreciable quantities of sympathomimetic amines. The reaction has been associated classically with tyramine, a natural byproduct of bacterial fermentation processes and found in many foods. Other aromatic amines can induce similar responses as a result of their ability to release norepinephrine from sympathetic nerve terminals. These indirectly sympathomimetic amines are usually cleared from the portal blood by the liver, but are not inactivated by deamination when MAO is inhibited. In addition to foods containing tyramine-like pressor amines, a large number of prescription drugs and proprietary medications contain sympathomimetic agents or other compounds that can induce untoward reactions in the presence of an MAO inhibitor. A partial list of commonly encountered foods to be avoided or eaten with caution includes: many cheeses (especially cheddars, Swiss, and Stilton) and, less importantly, yogurt; many alcoholic beverages (generally beer and wine, but particularly chianti); almost any product made with yeast or by bacterial action; canned fish products; snails; chopped liver; certain fruits, nuts, and vegetables (notably broad beans, which contain dopa, and citrus fruits and their juices, which contain tyramine); large quantities of coffee; and possibly cream and chocolate and food products prepared from them. Realistically, because more than 10 mg of tyramine is required to produce hypertension, the most likely foods are the cheeses and certain yeast products used as food supplements. Medications to be avoided or used cautiously include the amphetamines and sympathomimetic phenylalkylamines: Benzedrine, Dexedrine, methamphetamine (Desoxyn), ephedrine, norephedrine, and phenylephrine (Neo-synephrine), some of which occur in proprietary cold and sinus medications and decongestant inhalers. Because L-dopa and alpha-methyldopa (Aldomet) are converted to sympathomimetic amines, they must also be avoided. Patients with pheochromocytoma or carcinoid syndrome should not receive an MAO inhibitor. Moreover, the combination of an MAO inhibitor with reserpine, guanethidine, or other agents with acute amine-releasing effects can also induce paradoxical hypertensive reactions and CNS excitation. If such a hypertensive reaction is encountered, the specific treatment is immediate but slow intravenous injection of a potent alpha-adrenergic blocking agent, such as phentolamine (Regitine) in doses of 5 mg as needed. In an emergency, if a specific alpha-blocking agent is not at hand, parenteral injections of chlorpromazine (Thorazine), 50 to 100 mg intramuscularly, can be used while appropriate medical treatment is arranged.

MAO inhibitors also produce unwanted *interactions with other medications* (Table 16). They potentiate many central depressants, including the barbiturates, minor tranquilizers, phenothiazines, antihistamines, narcotic analgesics, and alcohol. *Meperidine* (Demerol) in particular has been associated with severe reactions that are not well understood pharmacologically; these include states of extreme excitement, seizures, and fever, as well as reactions resembling overdoses of a narcotic, even coma. *Narcotics* should *never* be used for headache in patients taking an MAO inhibitor, and the *headache* requires immediate evaluation of blood pressure. MAO inhibitors require particular caution in the management of surgical anesthesia, and they should be avoided for at least several days prior to surgery. The combination of an MAO inhibitor and a tricyclic antidepressant can, as was mentioned above, induce severe reactions. These include hypertensive crises, central excitation, seizures, hyperpyrexia, and death, especially when parenteral or high doses of the tricyclic agents are used. The demethylated tricyclic antidepressants, as selective and potent blockers of norepinephrine uptake, are particularly likely to produce *hyper*tension with an MAO inhibitor. Potentiation of anticholinergic or antiparkinson agents, oral hypoglycemics, and insulin by MAO inhibitors can also be anticipated. MAO inhibitors in combination with salt-losing diuretic agents have induced severe *hypo*tension. It should also be realized that some drugs other than antidepressants have MAO-inhibiting effects. These include the antihypertensive agent pargyline (Eutonyl), the nitrofuran antibiotics such as furazolidone (Furoxone), and a cancer-chemotherapy agent procarbazine (Matulane).

Stimulant drugs, and especially the amphetamines were formerly used in the attempt to treat depression, often in combination with barbiturates for anxiety and agitation. The most common stimulants now in use are amphetamines: *d, l-*

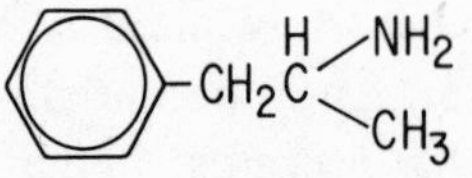

Amphetamine (Benzedrine, Dexedrine)

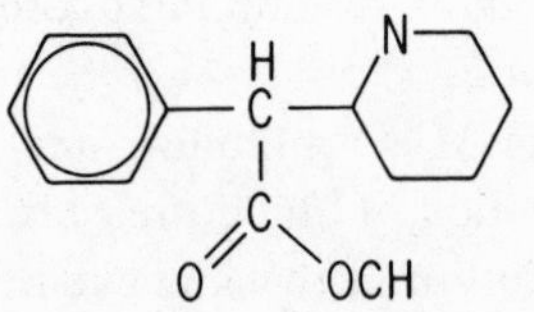

Methylphenidate (Ritalin)

Figure 8. Stimulants

amphetamine (Benzedrine), *d*-amphetamine (Dexedrine), and methamphetamine (Methedrine, Desoxyn, and others); and methylphenidate (Ritalin) (Figure 8, Table 17). These agents have peripheral and central sympathomimetic effects, potentiate the availability and activity of catecholamines, and produce strong cortical arousal, probably through brainstem mechanisms mediated by the ascending reticular activating system. They usually induce behavioral-activating or euphoriant effects, but in some subjects occasionally induce somnolence or dysphoria.

Their cortical arousal actions evidently underlie their usefulness in the management of the rare neurological syndrome, *narcolepsy*, for which antidepressants are also helpful, and may contribute to their well demonstrated usefulness in the childhood syndrome known as hyperactivity or "minimal brain dysfunction" (Table 18). The mechanisms by which amphetamines and other stimulants affect hyperactive children are not fully understood. One hypothesis is that these are "paradoxical" actions of stimulants on the immature or abnormal nervous system. It is more likely that the effects are mediated by normal mechanisms of increased cortical arousal that permit maximal attention and selective inhibition of behavior, and that these effects are only apparently paradoxical. The stimulants are not used with psychotic, autistic, or brain-damaged children, as increased excitement, agitation, or paranoid reactions may develop with these agents. Stimulants may induce tics in some children.

Stimulants also have some short-lasting anorexic effects, but after the initial few days of dieting are not useful for weight

Table 18. Stimulants and Related Agents for Hyperactivity or Minimal Brain Dysfunction ("MBD") in Children, and Dosages[a]

Agent	Typical Daily Dose (mg)	Dose Range (mg)
d-Amphetamine (Dexedrine, generic)	10–40 (0.5–1 mg/kg)	5–80 (0.2–3 mg/kg)
Methylphenidate (Ritalin)	30–80 (1–2 mg/kg)	10–150 (0.5–5 mg/kg)
Mg-Pemoline (Cylert)	50–100 (2–3 mg/kg)	25–125 (1–5 mg/kg)
Imipramine (Tofranil)	75–150 (2–4 mg/kg)	25–200 (25–200 mg/kg)

a. These agents are used most commonly between ages 6 and 16, and are useful for hyperactive and distractable patients who are *not* brain-damaged, retarded, autistic or psychotic. d,1-Amphetamine (Benzedrine, etc.) is as effective as d-amphetamine in similar doses, as was 1-amphetamine, given experimentally. Generally d-amphetamine or methylphenidate are started at 2.5 or 5.0 mg at breakfast or breakfast plus lunch, and gradually increased to an effective dose. Pemoline can be given as a single morning dose. Imipramine is almost certainly effective for MBD, and may also help childhood enuresis in doses of 25–75 mg at bedtime. Deanol (Deaner) and caffeine may be effective in MBD but are not as well established. Neuroleptic and antianxiety agents are not used in the MBD syndrome and lithium is ineffective.

control except for their placebo effect. Similarly, they have consistently been poor and ineffective antidepressants in controlled studies. Stimulants as well as the catecholamine precursor L-dopa, which has been tried as an experimental therapy for depression, may induce or increase psychotic agitation in severe depression. It is sometimes claimed that stimulants have something to offer in the management of short-lived neurotic forms of depressive illness, although this is a questionable indication, for which psychosocial interventions are usually appropriate.

Thus, psychiatric indications for the use of amphetamines in practice are very limited. Moreover, there is a considerable risk of abuse of this class of agents. Although the risk of true physiological addiction is often exaggerated, dysphoria and depression of mood ("crashing") commonly follow the abrupt discontinuation of high doses of amphetamines. In very high and prolonged doses, amphetamines and other stimulants, including cocaine, can induce a paranoid psychosis responsive to antipsychotic drugs, and in lower doses they can induce psychotic exacerbations in schizophrenic patients. Since they are such ineffective antidepressants and poor anorexic agents, it is remarkable that their production and prescription continue at excessively high rates.

Summary

The modern chemotherapy of depression is based on the use of a series of nonplanar structural analogues of the phenothiazines. In contrast to the largely antiadrenergic antipsychotic agents, these "tricyclic" antidepressants potentiate the actions of catecholamines; they also have strong antimuscarinic effects. The latter actions contribute to their annoying and more serious atropine-like effects on the eye, salivary glands, heart, gut, bladder, and central nervous system. It is unfortunate that the drugs used for patients at increased risk of suicide are so toxic and potentially lethal. While antidepressant effects of the tricyclic antidepressants have been demonstrated in controlled clinical trials among outpatients as well as inpatients, their efficacy is more impressive in the more severe forms of depression. For milder forms of the syndrome, their effects are not much better than those of antianxiety agents, a placebo or other nonspecific treatments, nor are they impressively better than psychotherapy. Even in serious depressions, the antidepressant drugs are usually not effective for a week or more after treatment is begun, and the rate of relapse is high unless patients are maintained on the medications for at least several months. In very severe cases of depression, more consistent and more rapid effects are obtained with ECT, which should still be used in the treatment of many very severe depressions, with acutely suicidal patients, and when the tricyclic antidepressants fail to work within a month or so, as happens in as many as 30% of severe depressions. The antipsychotic agents are also useful in the treatment of agitated and psychotic forms of depression. The MAO inhibitors are now largely of historical interest. With the exception of tranylcypromine, and possibly also phenelzine in high doses, they are inferior antidepressants and their use is complicated by many restrictions resulting from their toxic interactions with other agents. Stimulants have little if any place in the treatment of serious depressive illnesses. Several experimental chemotherapies for depression have been investigated, including a number of hormones and precursors of biogenic amines, but have not resulted in useful treatments. Owing to the limited efficacy, slowness and toxicity of the currently available agents, the search for better antidepressants must be pursued. There has been nothing fundamentally new in the treatment of depression since the introduction of ECT in the 1930s and the MAO inhibitors and imipramine in the 1950s.

5. Antianxiety Drugs

There is no ideal generic term for this class of agents. Use of the synonyms "antianxiety," "anxiolytic," or "tranquilizer" to some degree represents wishful thinking based on a long search for drugs that are specific for anxiety and distinctly different from the sedatives, hypnotics, and general anesthetics. Antianxiety agents have been of interest to physicians throughout the history of medicine. A hundred years ago, the main antianxiety agents were the bromide salts and ethanol administered as self medication, in patent remedies, or by prescription. With the development of pharmaceutical technology in the late nineteenth and early twentieth centuries, several compounds similar to alcohol were added, including paraldehyde and chloral hydrate. Then the barbiturates, of which at least fifty reached clinical use, soon became the standard sedatives and hypnotics. More recently the use of propanediols was initiated by the description in 1946 of the muscle-relaxant and sedative properties of the impractically short-acting agent mephenesin. In 1951, B. Ludwig and E. Piech produced meprobamate (Miltown, Equanil), a structural analogue of mephenesin with more prolonged muscle-relaxant and sedative actions, demonstrated by F. Berger in 1954. Meprobamate was shown to be useful in anxious patients by N. Dixon in 1957. Since then, other propanediols, including tybamate (Solacen, Tybatran), have been developed (Table 19). The search for safer antianxiety agents lacking addictive and other potentially lethal properties —central depression, respiratory depression—of all of the previously mentioned sedative-hypnotic tranquilizing agents led to the development of the benzodiazepines. While this latter class of chemicals had been known at least since the 1930s, with the ferment in psychopharmacology of the 1950s their reinvestigation led to the synthesis and study by L. Sternbach of chlordiazepoxide (Librium), which was introduced in 1960. It was found to have potent taming effects in animals and anticonvulsant, skeletal-muscle relaxant, and sedative-anti-anxiety effects in man. Since then, a number of structural variants of chlordiazepoxide have been introduced (Figure 9, Table 20). The enormous popularity of the benzodiazepines is illustrated by the fact that in the past several years diazepam (Valium) and chlordiazepoxide (Librium) have been among the *most prescribed* drugs of *all* kinds, at rates approaching 100 million prescriptions a year in the United States and a cost of about 500 million dollars! Another benzodiazepine, flurazepam (Dalmane), is one of the safest and most widely used sedative-hypnotics. The benzodiazepines are popular because they have significant antianxiety effects and are relatively safe. Despite their popularity, they and sedative-tranquilizing agents in general have been severely criticized in recent years. Too often, they are used in an allopathic compulsion to give something to ease the patient's pain, and as a substitute for the time required to assist an anxious or unhappy patient to discover and modify the source of psychic pain.

A limiting factor in the discovery and development of new antianxiety agents is the same as with preclinical pharmacological identification of potential antipsychotic agents by their neuroleptic effects and antidepressants by their adrenergic potentiating effects. With the anxiolytic sedatives, the animal

SEDATIVE-ANTIANXIETY AGENTS

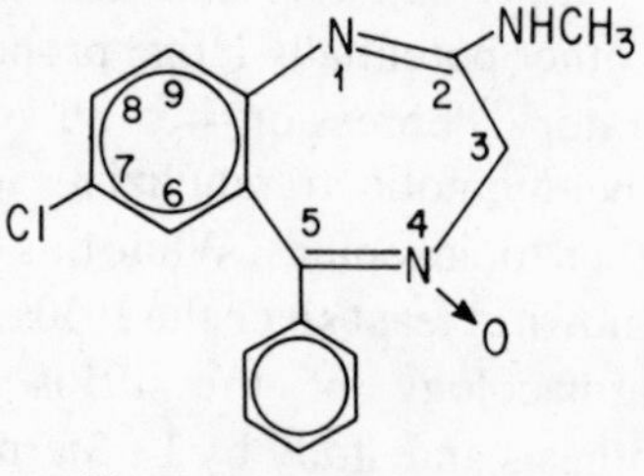

Chlordiazepoxide
(Librium)

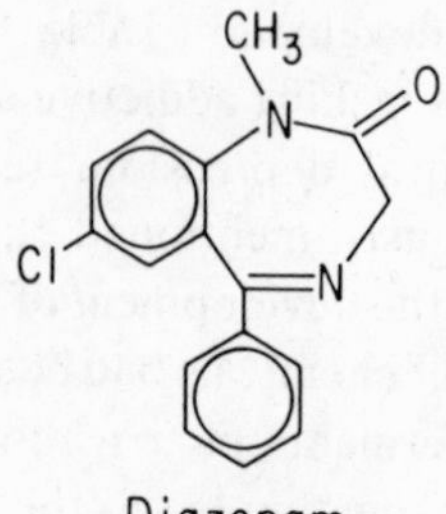

Diazepam
(Valium)

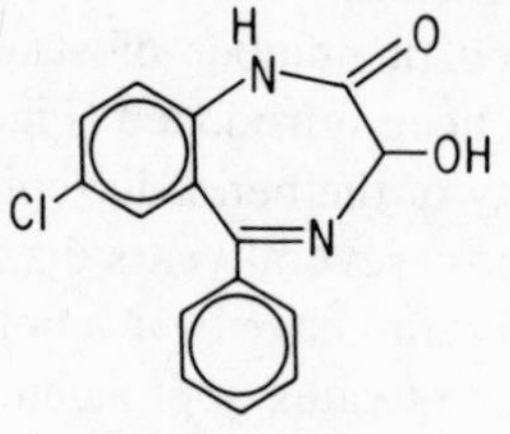

Oxazepam
(Serax)

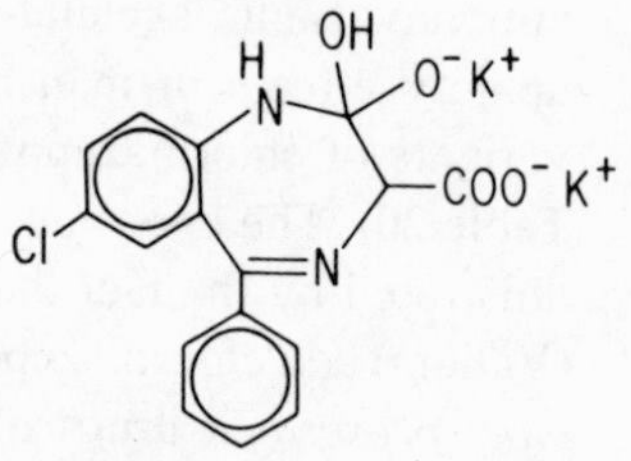

Chlorazepate
(Tranxene)

SEDATIVE-HYPNOTICS

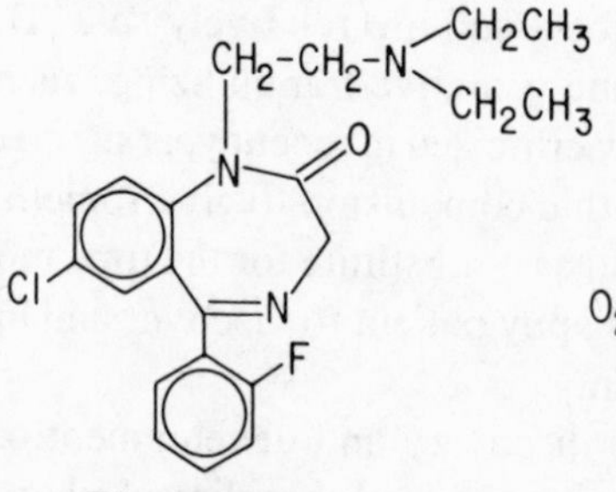

Flurazepam
(Dalmane)

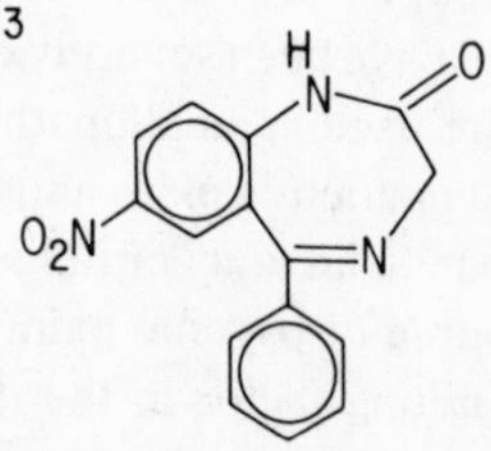

Nitrazepam
(Mogodon)

Figure 9. Benzodiazepine sedative-tranquilizers and hypnotics tests commonly used are those developed through experience with the barbiturates and include decreases in spontaneous and conditioned responses, increased seizure threshold, production of ataxia, and the prolongation and potentiation of sedative effects of a standard barbiturate. Experimental treatments of anxiety include the use of beta-adrenergic blocking agents such as propranolol (Inderal) that prevent many of the peripheral autonomic expressions of anxiety and stress.

Pharmacology

The sedative agents used to treat anxiety and mild dysphoria all depress the CNS, approximately in proportion to the dose. Milder central depression can provide clinically useful antianxiety effects more or less distinct from frank sedation. Many sedative agents also have anticonvulsant actions presumably secondary to depression of cortical neurons. Furthermore, muscle-relaxant properties are particularly evident with the propanediols and the benzodiazepines, either as a direct effect on skeletal muscles or because reflexes are blocked at the spinal cord level. Larger amounts of sedatives result in a gradually increasing toxic brain syndrome similar to intoxication with alcohol; still larger amounts result in profound central depression and eventually in coma, respiratory depression and death. Important related characteristics, shared to some degree by all of the sedative-tranquilizers, including the benzodiazepines, are their tendency to be required in increasing doses due to behavioral and pharmacodynamic *tolerance,* and their potential for producing psychological and physical dependence and *addiction.* Trends in the historical development of these agents have included a gradual improvement of their therapeutic indices and consequent separation of antianxiety and sedative effects, and a lessening of their addictive potential, most notably with the benzodiazepines. Most

sedative-antianxiety agents have relatively little effect on autonomic functions such as blood pressure, little ability to antagonize catecholamines and acetylcholine, and very little effect on
the extrapyramidal system—all in contrast to the antipsychotic agents. Exceptional are the more "antiautonomic" sedatives, including the antihistaminic compounds such as diphenhydramine (Benadryl) and hydroxyzine (Atarax, Vistaril).
The sedative-tranquilizers do not have useful antipsychotic
activity.

The barbiturates (Table 19) continue to be used by some
physicians for the management of neurotic anxiety and dysphoria. Phenobarbital is the most commonly used. It is a
long-acting barbiturate and is to a considerable degree excreted by the kidney (20–30%) independent of its hepatic
metabolism; in contrast, the shorter-acting barbiturates are
more rapidly metabolized, almost entirely by hepatic enzy-
matic activity. Thus, phenobarbital can be used cautiously in
small doses even in patients with liver disease; it can be used in
renal failure, too, although its actions will be prolonged. The
difficulty of obtaining a quick subjective "high" with phenobarbital decreases its potential for abuse, and its prolonged
duration of action reduces its ability to produce severe withdrawal reactions. On the other hand, the drug's persistence
complicates the management of potentially lethal acute overdoses. Phenobarbital can induce synthesis and activity of hepatic microsomal enzymes, and thus its own rate of metabolism, although this effect is not believed to be an important
factor in the production of tolerance to the barbiturates. However, it can have important consequences for the actions of
other drugs and hormones, including increased *inactivation* of
dihydroxycoumarin and steroids, and increased production of
porphyrins (Table 16).

The propanediols (Table 19) are metabolized mainly by hepatic microsomal oxidases, and meprobamate shares with the

Table 19. Sedatives

Generic Name	Trade Name	Comments
Alcohols, aldehydes and propanediols		
Ethanol	generic	not recommended[a]
Ethchlorvynol	Placidyl	not recommended[a]
Chloral hydrate	generic	1–2 gm for sleep
Paraldehyde	generic	not recommended[a]
Meprobamate	Equanil, Miltown, generic	not recommended[a]
Tybamate	Tybatran, Solacen, generic	not recommended[a]
Barbiturates		
Amobarbital	Amytal, generic	100–800 mg/hr, intravenously in diagnosis, or parenterally for emergency sedation
Methohexital	Brevital	10 mg/5 sec intravenously for ECT only
Pentobarbital	Nembutal, generic	can be used for withdrawal in most sedative addictions[b,c]
Phenobarbital	Luminal, generic	30–90 mg/day[b,c]
Secobarbital	Seconal, generic	not recommended[b]
Structural relatives of barbiturates (nonbarbiturates)		
Glutethimide	Doriden	not recommended[a]
Methyprylon	Noludar	not recommended[a]
Methaqualone	Quaalude, Sopor, generic	not recommended[a]
Antihistamines		
Diphenhydramine	Benadryl	25–50 mg parenterally for dystonia[d]
Hydroxyzine	Atarax, Vistaril	not recommended[a]
Promethazine	Phenergan, generic	not recommended[a]

a. Some agents are not recommended for routine use as sedatives.

b. Sometimes short-acting barbiturates, while not generally recommended are used for sleep because of their low cost; phenobarbital is a very inexpensive sedative and not often abused.

c. Pentobarbital and phenobarbital are often used to treat addiction to this entire class of agents; see Table 21.

d. Diphenhydramine and other antihistamines are sometimes used as sedatives in pediatric practice.

barbiturates their ability to induce these enzymes. Because meprobamate is more rapidly excreted than phenobarbital (half-life, about twelve hours for meprobamate versus more than twenty-four hours for phenobarbital), an increased rate of oxidation probably contributes to tolerance of this drug. Tybamate is even more rapidly metabolized and excreted than meprobamate; so its useful duration of action is also less by about 50%, but also the probability of physiological addiction is reduced because much less drug accumulates in tissue. True physical addiction to meprobamate is well known and can occur after prolonged use of doses not much greater than the upper limits of recommended doses.

The benzodiazepines (Figure 9, Table 20) have become extraordinarily popular in the past decade. Initially they were thought to be pharmacologically dissimilar to other sedatives. In fact, however, this class of agents is in many respects qualitatively similar to the older sedatives, including the barbiturates and the propanediols. Thus, the benzodiazepines have widespread, diffuse inhibitory effects in the CNS and important anticonvulsant activity as well as muscle-relaxant activity, partly mediated by inhibitory effects on reflex activity, especially on polysynaptic reflexes at the spinal cord and at higher levels. The benzodiazepines, like nearly all of the sedatives, produce slow wave and low-voltage, fast (beta) activity in the EEG.

The benzodiazepines do have characteristics that separate them from the barbiturates and are partially shared by the propanediols. These include depression of the limbic system (especially the septum, amygdala, and hippocampus) at lower doses than more generalized depression of the cerebral cortex and the reticular activating system. This partial selectivity correlates with taming effects in animals and the suppression of conditional (especially "avoidance" behaviors) more than unconditional responses in animals. In man, the selective action of the benzodiazepines is manifested in an antianxiety effect relatively free of the sedation and mental clouding typical of older sedatives.

Most of the sedative-tranquilizers (except the antihistamines) exhibit *cross-tolerance,* the ability of one to induce tolerance to the effects of the others. This observation supports the conclusion that the actions of all of these agents are similar. A practical consequence of cross-tolerance is that withdrawal of addicting doses of any of these agents can be accomplished by the use of gradually diminishing doses of any one of them; commonly a barbiturate is used. The benzodiazepines, like all of the sedative-tranquilizing agents, are limited by the development of tolerance to their main or desired antianxiety effect as well as to the degree of sedation they produce. This aspect of their actions limits the length of time they are clinically useful and contributes to their abuse. In addition to tolerance, almost all of the drugs employed to treat anxiety—barbiturates, propanediols and other nonbarbiturate sedatives, and benzodiazepines—but not the less frequently used antihistamines, produce true physiological dependence and significant withdrawal syndromes on abrupt discontinuation of high doses. However, the benzodiazepines are less likely to produce dangerous withdrawal syndromes, and are unlikely to produce even mild withdrawal after less than two months of use. The danger of severe coma, respiratory depression and death following an acute overdose of a benzodiazepine is also less than after a comparable multiple of the average daily dose of a barbiturate, propanediol or other sedative. One way of summarizing the unique characteristics of the benzodiazepines is to point out that their dose-response relationships are much "flatter" than those of the barbiturates and nonbarbiturate sedatives (but less gradual than those of the antipsychotic agents), so that doubling the dose produces proportionally less sedation than occurs with the other sedatives.

The benzodiazepines (Figure 9) differ one from another in pharmacokinetics and metabolism. Diazepam (Valium) is rapidly absorbed after oral administration; its speed of action and greater potency contribute to its ability to induce euphoria and acute intoxication and thus to its recent popularity as a drug of abuse. Diazepam is one of the most lipophilic benzodiazepines, with a marked tendency to accumulate in tissues and to undergo prolonged elimination. Its half-life in man is several days, in contrast to 8–15 hours for oxazepam (Serax) and 12–24 hours for chlordiazepoxide (Librium). The binding of diazepam to membranes and plasma proteins makes it relatively difficult to remove by diuresis or dialysis after acute overdoses.

Like tricyclic antidepressants, some benzodiazepines can be converted to active, and sometimes clinically useful metabolites. Benzodiazepines are metabolized by hepatic microsomal enzymes to oxidized and demethylated products which are mainly conjugated with glucuronic acid prior to their removal in the urine and feces. Chlordiazepoxide forms two major metabolites. In one the amino methyl is removed and in the other a keto oxygen replaces the side amino group entirely to make a metabolite resembling diazepam; both metabolites have sedative activity. Similarly, diazepam is metabolized first to a demethylated form, and thence to oxazepam (Serax); both metabolites have biological activity, although oxazepam does not remain in the blood or tissue long enough to contribute importantly to the overall activity of diazepam and its demethylated product. Chlorazepate (Tranxene) is probably not an active substance *in vivo,* as it is rapidly transformed to demethyldiazepam, and only this metabolite is found in the blood; the active metabolite is known to accumulate in tissues and to undergo slow excretion, much as diazepam does.

Flurazepam (Dalmane) and nitrazepam (Mogodon) are much more like sedatives than the other benzodiazepines in that their "antianxiety" or behavior-inhibiting effects in animals are produced at doses very close to those that induce ataxia and somnolence; consequently their current main use is as hypnotic agents. *In vivo,* flurazepam is rapidly converted to a more slowly cleared, active metabolite by removal of its side chain. Development of tolerance to sedation by flurazepam is much less than with other hypnotics. Although the benzodiazepines can induce hepatic enzymes, this mechanism is generally not significant. It does not contribute appreciably to increased tolerance of the benzodiazepines, and because it does not increase the inactivation rate of other drugs, such as the coumarin anticoagulants or the antidepressants, increased doses of those drugs are not required as they would be in association with the barbiturates and glutethimide.

Clinical Use

None of the sedative-tranquilizer group of antianxiety drugs is useful as a primary therapeutic agent in severe psychiatric illness, although they have occasional applications in such patients. The main usefulness of the antianxiety agents is in the *short-term* treatment of relatively transient forms of anxiety, fear, and tension. They are also widely used as preoperative sedatives, in the management of short-lived painful syndromes, and in psychosomatic and other illnesses with unexplained physical manifestations. Benzodiazepines have been claimed to have some immediate euphoriant and antianxiety effects in moderately severe anxious neurotic depressions, and to be of some benefit during the delayed onset of action of an antidepressant. The development of tolerance to the antianxiety, euphoriant, and sedative effects of all sedative-tranquilizers results in a loss of their clinical effectiveness over time and contributes to an increased risk of dependency, abuse, and addiction. Many psychiatrists believe that pro-

longed nonpsychotic disorders involving anxiety and dysphoria are better treated with psychotherapy, and limit antianxiety agents to brief use in the less common, more acute,
short-lived, and usually reactive forms of neurotic illness.
Their prolonged use in the management of neurotic psychiatric
illnesses that overlap with the chronic characterological disorders is even less satisfactory. Consequently, these agents
are more often used in general medicine than in psychiatry.

The usefulness of this class of agents is optimized by careful
attention to subtleties of their actions and of the doctor-patient
relationship. Many psychotherapists are particularly disin-
clined to rely on the antianxiety agents inasmuch as the descrip-
tive characteristics of patients who respond well to antianxiety
agents differ from those of patients usually considered good
candidates for the rational and verbal psychotherapies. Thus, a
favorable response has been associated with relatively lower
socioeconomic class, lack of psychological sophistication, and
inability to express unhappiness verbally in terms of intrapsychic or interpersonal conflict. A more favorable response
also occurs in patients with passive and almost magical
expectations of the physician. An enthusiastic, charismatic
presentation of the medication and its effects by the physician
seems to be helpful. Patients who are active, vigorous, and
extroverted tend to dislike the sedative effects of antianxiety
agents, and may even become more uncomfortable taking
them.

The broad and loosely defined applications of antianxiety
agents severely complicate the interpretation of data based on
even their well designed, controlled clinical trials. The rate of
favorable responses to a placebo in many of these trials has
ranged from 20 or 30% to as much as 60% depending on the
group of patients. This variability of patient selection and the
strong placebo effect make it difficult to demonstrate significant benefits of an active antianxiety drug. Benefits of medica-

tion are particularly difficult to demonstrate in short-lived, reactive forms of anxiety that improve even without chemical interventions. The main conclusions based on several extensive reviews of clinical drug trials are that sedative-tranquilizing agents do have appreciable and fairly consistent antianxiety effects beyond those of a placebo, and that it is extremely difficult to demonstrate the superiority of one agent or class of agents over another. A specific agent must, then, be selected on the basis of considerations other than its demonstrated superiority in a given condition (Tables 19 and 20). For routine use in psychiatric patients, and indeed most patients, most of the short-acting *barbiturates and nonbarbiturate sedatives* should not be used for prolonged daytime sedation and antianxiety effects because of their potential for excessive sedation and their high addiction potential and overdose lethality. However, it is well to remember that the long-acting barbiturate phenobarbital has done about as well as the more modern antianxiety agents in most drug comparisons, and it is far less expensive. Although there is little reason to recommend short-acting barbiturates as antianxiety agents they still have specialized uses in psychiatry. For example, they (as well as diazepam or droperidol) are occasionally used in emergencies to produce rapid sedation in psychotic, manic, or enraged patients, usually in conjunction with a sedating antipsychotic agent such as chlorpromazine. Short-acting barbiturates, most commonly amobarbital, given intravenously are occasionally used to facilitate the differential diagnosis of catatonic behavior or in attempts to uncover highly defended thoughts or feelings in diagnostic sessions or abreactive therapeutic interviews.

The *propanediols,* which seemed promising in the 1950s are no better than the barbiturates, and meprobamate carries an unacceptable risk of addiction and fatality on overdosage. The addicting dose of meprobamate overlaps the therapeutic range:

physical signs of withdrawal can follow the discontinuation of doses as low as 1200 mg/day, and severe withdrawal and seizures can be expected at doses above 3200 mg/day, while the therapeutic range is 1200 to 2400 mg/day. A newer propanediol, tybamate, is much less likely to produce addiction, but comparisons with barbiturates and the benzodiazepines have shown it to be an inferior antianxiety agent.

The *benzodiazepines* (Table 20) have become so popular because their effects in anxiety are consistently superior to a placebo, and because they are relatively safe agents, to which it is difficult to become addicted and with which it is difficult to commit suicide. For reasons that are not entirely clear, diazepam (Valium) has become the most popular benzodiazepine in the 1970s; it outsells its closest rival, chlordiazepoxide (Librium), by more than two to one. The benzodiazepines are relatively expensive.

Unfortunately, the rapid activity of diazepam and its tendency to induce euphoria have made it a popular drug of abuse. Its prolonged duration of action and affinity for lipid and protein suggest that overdoses of diazepam may be somewhat more dangerous than those of other benzodiazepines. Oxazepam (Serax) is the most rapidly metabolized and cleared benzodiazepine; it has no active metabolites or tendency to accumulate in tissue. It may, then, be safer for use in elderly patients or those with impaired hepatic function. Oxazepam is also the most potent anticonvulsant of this group of drugs. Flurazepam (Dalmane) and nitrazepam (Mogodon), which is not available in the United States, are more potent in their sedative effects than the other benzodiazepines and are recommended only for nighttime sedation and sleep. They also seem to have less tendency to induce tolerance than other hypnotics. It is not yet clearly established, but their lethality on overdosage and potential for abuse and addiction appear to be no greater than for other benzodiazepines and much less than for

Table 20. Tranquilizing Sedatives Used for Anxiety: Benzodiazepines

Generic Name	Trade Name	Dose Range (mg/day)	Ratio of Lethal Dose[a] to Daily Dose
Sedative-tranquilizers			
Chlordiaz-epoxide	Librium, generic	15–100 (up to 400 mg in delirium tremens)	>10
Chlorazepate	Tranxene	15–60	> 5
Diazepam	Valium	6–40	>20
Oxazepam	Serax	30–120	?
Sedative-hypnotics			
Flurazepam	Dalmane	15–30 (at bedtime)	>10
Nitrazepam	(Mogodon)	unavailable in U. S.	?

a. The human lethal dose of the benzodiazepines is poorly established, but exceeds a week's supply of ordinary doses. Rare fatalities have been reported after 700–1000 mg of Librium or Valium.

the short-acting barbiturates and nonbarbiturate hypnotic-sedatives.

A specialized use of benzodiazepines is to control *acute toxic psychoses* brought on by *hallucinogenic* agents, such as lysergic acid diethylamide (LSD), methylated aromatic amines, or phencyclidine, that may occasionally produce unwanted drug interactions, including hypotension, when antipsychotic agents are given. Many milder cases, especially with LSD or mescaline, can be managed even more conservatively by protection and reassurance until the effects of the psychotogen wear off. The notable exception to this rule is the paranoid psychosis induced by large or prolonged doses of amphetamines; it responds quickly, specifically, and safely to antipsychotic agents, and is unnecessarily prolonged without such treatment.

In *elderly patients,* there is little reason to use barbiturates for agitation or insomnia. The risks of paradoxical excitement and increased agitation, intoxication, fatal overdosage, and complex drug interactions from induction of hepatic enzymes outweigh the beneficial effects of barbiturates and the related nonbarbiturate sedative agents. Although benzodiazepines are relatively safer, they too are sometimes associated with excessive sedation, intoxication, and occasionally, paradoxical excitation. Due to its rapid clearance, oxazepam may be particularly safe for use in elderly patients.

For *children,* barbiturates (and diphenylhydantoin) should only be used as anticonvulsants and not as sedatives or behavior-modifying agents. When a hypnotic effect is desirable or to calm severe acute excitement, diphenhydramine (Benadryl) is commonly used in doses from 50 to 500 mg/day (2–20 mg/kg), and chloral hydrate still has a useful place in doses from 500 to 2500 mg (up to 50 mg/kg). Information concerning the use of benzodiazepines for the control of anxiety and behavioral disorders in children is scant; chlordiazepoxide (Librium) is the best evaluated agent of this class. This drug is not as useful as amphetamine in the control of hyperactivity (Table 18). Chlordiazepoxide has been reported to have some beneficial effects, as have tricyclic and MAO inhibitor antidepressants, on phobic states including school phobias, in doses of 30–130 mg/day (1.0–5.0 mg/kg). There is probably an increased risk of paradoxical excitement and rage reactions when benzodiazepines are given to brain-damaged children or those with a history of aggressive or impulsive behavior.

Toxicity and Unwanted Effects

For all sedatives, the most commonly encountered problem is daytime sedation with drowsiness, decreased mental acuity, some decrease in coordination, decreased occupational productivity, and increased risk of accidents, particularly when sedatives are combined with alcohol. Autonomic and extrapyramidal side effects are not usually encountered with the sedatives. Liver damage and blood dyscrasias are rare. Sedatives can interact significantly with other medications; such interactions are particularly likely with the barbiturates, and rare with the benzodiazepines (Table 16).

It would be a mistake to conclude that the benzodiazepines are totally innocuous. In rare cases overdoses equivalent to about a 2 weeks' supply, or even less if taken with alcohol, have led to death. The common use of chlordiazepoxide and diazepam in high doses to treat alcoholic withdrawal and the use of diazepam intravenously to control seizures or cardiac arrhythmias, occasionally are complicated by apnea, ventricular arrhythmias, or cardiac arrest. Certain neurotic or psychotic patients, and even normal volunteers occasionally become dysphoric, agitated, angry, "touchy" or otherwise "disinhibited" while taking benzodiazepines. This effect resembles that of alcohol and, while most commonly ascribed to chlordiazepoxide, is not unique to that agent. Rarely, frank rage reactions have been observed.

The most serious problems of sedatives are related to their tendency to produce *tolerance* and physiological *addiction* in addition to psychological dependence. Moreover, in varying degrees they are lethal in acute overdoses. Tolerance to the antianxiety and sedative effects of sedatives can contribute to innocent self-medication in increasing doses. Rapid intoxication and euphoria from large or parenteral doses of the short-acting barbiturates, most of the nonbarbiturate sedative-hypnotics, and diazepam most impressively among the benzodiazepines contribute to their abuse and to a brisk black market in these agents.

It is currently a topic of debate whether the industrially developed societies of the world are "overmedicated," and particularly whether the current medical use of drugs to treat mild neurotic reactions and even "normal" stresses and strains of living contributes to the abuse of psychotropic agents. While the debate continues, physicians can deal with the problems associated with sedative-tranquilizing agents by selecting those with less potential for abuse, addiction, and lethality and by using the drugs for clear indications and for short periods of time. Patients with a previous history of abuse of other sedatives or alcohol and with other dyssocial or impulsive traits should be treated with this class of agents very cautiously. In general, the use of sedative-tranquilizers in patients with character disorders and more characterological forms of neurosis is unlikely to be helpful except in acute exacerbations of turmoil or anticipatory anxiety, and is likely to engender abuse.

The probability that a patient will become *physically addicted* to a sedative increases with the daily dose of drug and the duration of its use. Meprobamate is so highly addicting as to make its use in other than moderate doses for brief periods impractical. With short-acting barbiturates, some signs and symptoms of withdrawal can be expected after the intake of about four to five times the usual daily dose for more than a month, and severe withdrawal reactions, with hypotension, seizures, delirium tremens, and hallucinosis can be expected to occur two or three days after discontinuation of prolonged dosage more than five times the ordinary daily dose, and certainly above ten times this dose. The withdrawal syndrome is strikingly similar to that associated with alcohol. It is most important to realize that withdrawal from addiction to barbiturates and other sedatives is a serious and *life-threatening* medical problem, in contrast to withdrawal from narcotics, which is unpleasant, but almost never fatal. Special measures to be taken in managing sedative withdrawal are outlined in Table 21. Physical dependence on the benzodiazepines has been studied most extensively with the oldest agents of that group,

Table 21. Principles of Withdrawal in Addiction to Barbiturates and Other Sedatives

1. A short-acting barbiturate (e.g., pentobarbital, Nembutal) has similar actions ("cross-tolerance") to most of the sedative-tranquilizers in Table 19 (except the antihistamines, which rarely produce addiction) and can be used to withdraw from nonbarbiturates as well as all barbiturates, greatly simplifying the technique.

2. Withdrawal from barbiturate-type addiction (in contrast to opioid addiction) is a medically serious undertaking, best done in hospital and carried out *slowly* (especially with phenobarbital, glutethimide, and the benzodiazepines, although the withdrawal syndrome with benzodiazepines is rarely severe).

3. Estimate the amount of pentobarbital required to protect against withdrawal symptoms after initial intoxication has cleared by giving sufficient doses (usually 200–400 mg, preferably orally) in 4–6 hour intervals to induce *mild* intoxication (drowsiness, slurred speech, ataxia, incoordination, nystagmus) within an hour of each dose and to avoid prominent withdrawal symptoms, tremulousness and hypotension 4–6 hours after each dose. In a 24-hour period 800–2400 mg are typically required; up to 400 mg/day of pentobarbital can be discontinued abruptly.

4. Stabilization continues for 2–3 days for most barbiturates and nonbarbiturate sedatives. The daily dose is given in 4–6 portions. Owing to their tendency to produce severe withdrawal symptoms a week or more after withdrawal, a stabilization period of 7–10 days is recommended for phenobarbital, glutethimide and following abuse of the benzodiazepines in very large doses.

5. Withdraw (over approximately 10–20 days) by removing not more than 100 mg of pentobarbital per day and *only* after stabilization is attained (mild intoxication and minimal withdrawal signs during a 24-hour period) and maintained for the recommended number of days. If withdrawal signs develop, stop withdrawal until the signs disappear and resume at 50 mg per day.

6. As an alternative to step 5, some experts recommend substituting phenobarbital (long-acting), 30 mg for each 100 mg of pentobarbital during the stabilization period and withdrawing it at the rate of 30 mg/day.

7. The short-acting barbiturates are not useful in the management of withdrawal from opiates. Even though there is cross-tolerance between alcohol and barbiturates, detoxification of alcoholics is usually accomplished with benzodiazepines (chlordiazepoxide or diazepam). Addiction to meprobamate is often overcome by slow withdrawal of the offending agent by the same principles outlined above.

chlordiazepoxide and diazepam. Addiction is not likely unless abuses reach at least ten, and more likely twenty times the usual daily oral dose and continue for several months. This time can be shortened if the drugs are taken intravenously, as has sometimes been done with diazepam in its recent abuse as a "street drug." The ordinarily delayed development of addiction to benzodiazepines in part reflects the prolonged half-life of these agents, much as the long-acting barbiturate phenobarbital infrequently leads to physical dependence and a withdrawal syndrome. Furthermore, the onset of the withdrawal syndrome with the benzodiazepines, glutethimide (Doriden), and phenobarbital is considerably later than with either the short-acting barbiturates and sedatives (two to three days) or alcohol (three to five days), and is usually seen at four to eight days, but as long as two weeks after withdrawal. Even when a withdrawal syndrome is encountered after abuse of the benzodiazepines it is likely to be of only moderate intensity and is rarely associated with seizures. The development of psychological and physiological dependence on sedative-hypnotic agents represents a complex relationship between their pharmacology and sociological factors involved in their use. One study reported, curiously, that the use of antianxiety medication *decreased* when patients were allowed to set their own dosage schedule according to their needs, in contrast to fixed dosage determined by the prescribing physician. However, tolerance to the effects of this class of agents can encourage innocent increases in the amount of medication. These considerations add further support to the conclusion that they should be used only in acute anxiety and for brief periods and that prolonged "maintenance" with antianxiety agents should be avoided.

The benzodiazepines have a comfortable margin of safety in comparison with other sedatives. Nevertheless, although it is commonly said that suicide is virtually impossible with a benzodiazepine, most deliberate overdoses involve more than one agent, typically whatever the victim has at hand and can present complicated toxicologic crises that are difficult to manage. The problem is exacerbated when patients acquire a number of potentially lethal medications from more than one source or from a single physician over time. Some of the problem could be eliminated by requiring that patients empty their medicine chests and bring *all* their medications to the physician, who should take the responsibility for disposing of the unnecessary or outdated ones before a new psychotropic chemical is prescribed. It is difficult to recommend a specific benzodiazepine supply that can be safely dispensed, since there are rare reports of deaths following the acute ingestion of 600–1000 mg of chlordiazepoxide or diazepam, and reports of the survival of doses of more than 2000 mg. With other sedatives and hypnotics, as a general rule, the acute ingestion of ten days' supply at once will regularly produce severe intoxication, and may be lethal, and the ingestion of twenty times the daily or hypnotic dose is very likely to be fatal. Thus, even though fatality is less likely and more unpredictable with acute overdoses of the benzodiazepines than with other sedative-tranquilizers, it is unwise to dispense more than perhaps two weeks' supply of a benzodiazepine or a week's supply of other sedatives. Moreover, continuing the use of any of these drugs for more than a few weeks is unlikely to be effective.

The safety of sedative-tranquilizers in pregnancy is not established. There is some recent evidence that the benzodiazepines may be teratogenic, inasmuch as cleft lip and palate have been suggestively associated with the use of a benzodiazepine in the first trimester of pregnancy. The barbiturates can alter fetal hepatic metabolism and should be avoided. Claims have been made for the safety of meprobamate in pregnancy, but physiological dependence of the fetus to it or to barbiturate and nonbarbiturate sedatives can be expected.

Summary

Anxiety and dysphoria are ubiquitous human experiences. They are most effectively and appropriately treated with chemotherapy when they represent acute and severe symptoms of neurotic psychiatric illness or reactive or anticipatory features of medical or surgical illness. Antianxiety medications should be used for brief periods of time because of tolerance to their antianxiety and sedative effects and the risk of psychological dependence and even physical addiction. Routine and sustained use for psychiatric patients with characterological disorders is of questionable value and presents increased risk of abuse. The history of psychopharmacology has been marked by the partially successful search for more effective and less toxic antianxiety agents and included the replacement of alcohol and the bromides by the barbiturates in the early twentieth century and the later addition of nonbarbiturate sedatives, including the propanediols. All of these agents are severely toxic and potentially lethal when taken acutely in doses above ten times the usual daily dose and physically addicting when used for several months at doses only a few times above the daily dose. Withdrawal can be managed by the substitution of a short-acting barbiturate and its *slow* withdrawal. Since the 1960s, the benzodiazepines have become the most useful antianxiety agents with the widest margin of safety and much less potential for addiction. They also have useful hypnotic, anticonvulsant, and muscle-relaxant effects. The "metapharmacological" aspects of anxiolytic agents, including psychosocial characteristics of patients and physicians using them, contribute to their efficacy, which depends at least partly on suggestion and placebo effects.

6. Special Topics

Geriatric and Pediatric Psychopharmacology

Use of psychiatric chemotherapy in patients at the extremes of the age spectrum raises several considerations. Although *geriatric psychopharmacology* remains a relatively underdeveloped area of investigation, the elderly represent an increasingly large proportion of psychiatric patients, partly as a reflection of their increased representation in the population. Between 1900 and 1970 the rate of increase of persons over age sixty-five was about seven times greater than that of the total population, so now elderly citizens of the United States exceed twenty million. Among elderly nursing home residents, 90% or more are estimated to have clinically significant neuropsychiatric disabilities and about 75% of these receive psychotropic medications. Many specific aspects of the use of antipsychotic, antidepressant, or antianxiety agents in the elderly have already been discussed.

In addition, attempts have been made to develop chemical treatments of the loss of cerebral function that is characteristic of advanced age. Thus, a special application of psychopharmacology in aged patients is the use of mild stimulants and putative cerebral vasodilators in an effort to improve senile mentation. Stimulants such as amphetamine or methylphenidate (Ritalin) often induce agitation and unwanted side effects in elderly patients. However, vasodilators such as papaverine (Pavabid), cyclandelate (Cyclospasmol), isoxuprene (Vasodilan), and hexobendine (investigational), ergot alkaloids (especially Hydergine), and beta-adrenergic blocking agents such as propranolol (Inderal) have all been claimed to produce improvement in behavior, mood and cortical functions. While these agents have some promise, their effectiveness is not well established by rigorously controlled studies. Some of these agents, as well as procainamide preparations (such as the European drug Gerovital), may also have euphoriant properties. Pemoline (Cylert) might also increase intellectual function, but its efficacy is not well established. All drugs of this type probably have placebo effects in addition to any specific pharmacologic activity they may possess.

There are several physiological characteristics of elderly patients that contribute to an increased risk of severe *toxic effects* of all medications. Patients in their seventies and eighties have been reported to have side effects due to many drugs two to three times more frequently than patients in their forties, and up to seven times more than patients in their twenties; adverse reactions occur in at least 25% of patients over eighty years old treated with medications of all kinds. The most common untoward effects are lethargy, confusion, and disorientation, or restlessness, agitation, and aggression; hypotension; urinary retention and ileus; and diminution of respiration. These reactions are particularly likely with drugs that act on the central nervous system, such as antipsychotic and antidepressant agents and sedative-tranquilizers. In elderly subjects the absorption, distribution, metabolism, and excretion of many drugs are decreased. An increased ratio of fat to lean body mass increases the retention of many centrally active drugs, including antipsychotic and antidepressant agents.

There may be an increased sensitivity to exogenous adrenergic agents. Generally, with advancing age there is a decreasing dosage requirement (or, more precisely, *decreased tolerance*), and a narrowing of the therapeutic index. At the other end of the age range, *pediatric psychopharmacology*, like geriatric psychopharmacology, is an underdeveloped area, marked by less rigor and fewer controlled trials of medications than exist for adults. There are a number of reasons for this situation. Differential diagnosis and even the classification of childhood mental illness are much less firmly established than for adults. The models of illness developed in adult psychiatry are not readily adapted to childhood, as children tend to respond with alterations of behavior or development, such as irritability, temper tantrums, hyperactivity, aggressiveness, withdrawal, regression, negativism, misbehavior or "acting-up," poor school performance, intellectual deterioration or slow development. Such reactions are much more typical than classical forms of thought disorder, depression, or mania which are seen in adults. For example, the term "schizophrenia" when applied to children is used very loosely, and has different meanings in various centers. Similar signs and symptoms can be associated with a wide range of problems: for example, minimal brain dysfunction, gross brain pathology, retardation, aphasia, autism, sensory deficits, functional psychosis, neglect, or environmental turmoil have many similar features. Another factor apparently contributing to the underdevelopment of pediatric psychopharmacology is that many psychiatrists interested in children have been strongly committed to psychosocial and developmental concepts in their therapeutic strategies. There is also a general tendency for adults to be protective of children, to be conservative about permitting the investigation of new therapies for them, and to be suspicious of medications that alter behavior or that may diminish intellectual, physical or social skills.

Outpatient Psychiatric Chemotherapy

There are general features of chemotherapy in an outpatient psychiatric setting that are somewhat different from those in a more controlled inpatient setting, and that require further consideration. Outpatient treatment including chemotherapy has become increasingly important since the 1950s in preventing hospitalization and in providing long-term care following hospitalization of seriously ill psychiatric patients, particularly since chemotherapy has its greatest impact with more severe illnesses.

A crucial aspect of outpatient practice involving medications is the patient's *cooperation* at the initiation of treatment and during the sometimes prolonged medical regimen required. Outpatient and inpatient psychiatric services differ in the degree to which the patient collaborates in the planning and execution of his treatment program. In the outpatient setting, it is the *patient,* and not the staff, who ultimately *controls* the decision to accept medication, ordinarily administers the medication, and is usually the first to detect beneficial or unwanted effects of a drug. Since the patient's cooperation is required, the routine and indifferent prescription of a medical treatment, particularly by a physician who may not know the patient well, and may not follow his progress by close personal contact, will have little chance of success even if the right drug is prescribed at the optimal dose as already outlined in previous chapters, particularly if the patient is depressed, confused or suspicious. Thus, considerable sensitivity and diplomacy are required to elicit the patient's informed cooperation. An authoritarian approach to medication may occasionally be warranted in an outpatient setting, for example when attempting to interrupt a psychotic or acute depressive illness that might otherwise require hospitalization or end in suicide. Generally, however, a flexible, open-minded, "advisory" attitude will more often lead to the acceptance of a medical regimen. A goal should be to encourage the development of positive feelings to the person most directly involved with the patient's care, and not to rely on exaggerated expectations of the efficacy of the chemotherapy. In that way, a cooperative working relationship can develop, and there is a greater likelihood that medication will be accepted, that minor side-effects will be tolerated, and that necessary modifications in the treatment can be made efficiently. The alternative is a dissatisfied and inadequately treated patient who may decline further care and encourage dissatisfaction and resentment in other patients.

It is important to provide for the outpatient and his family detailed information and *education* about the use of medications so they can arrive at informed consent to the treatment. In an outpatient setting, such information may be even more crucial than on an acute inpatient service, particularly when potentially toxic and expensive drugs must be used for prolonged periods, or even indefinitely. It is not only more humane and legally wise to practice chemotherapy in this manner, but it will also improve the safety of treatment, by encouraging earlier recognition of drug side-effects, and will contribute to a relationship between patient and doctor that is more likely to endure. Some clinicians provide and discuss written lists of specific warnings about the symptoms of drug toxicity, the description and dosage of medication, and conditions that might represent increased medical risks to patients. Some points to be included in such an approach are suggested in Table 22. It is possible to attend to these matters without being unnecessarily alarming, and since some side effects are common, it is unrealistic and misleading to avoid discussing them. At times when a patient is too confused, suspicious or depressed to manage his own medication safely, a family member may be instructed about the effects of a drug and given responsibility for storing and dispensing it.

Table 22. Information to Elicit Regularly about Drug Side Effects

Antipsychotic agents

- Sedation, "depression"
- Dry mouth, blurred vision, constipation, urinary hesitation
- Restlessness, muscle spasms, awkwardness, sluggishness, shaking
- Itching, color of urine, stool and skin, sun sensitivity
- Sore throat, malaise, fever
- Pregnancy
- Sexual dysfunction

Lithium

- Following prescription and blood testing protocols exactly
- Nausea, vomiting, diarrhea, metallic taste
- Trembling, awkwardness, unsteadiness, confusion (especially in the elderly)
- Thirst, urinary frequency
- Enlargement of thyroid
- Skin rashes
- Pregnancy

Antidepressants

- Sedation, confusion (especially in the elderly)
- Dry mouth, vile taste, blurred vision, urinary hesitation, constipation
- Other medications used
- Skin rashes, sunburn, color of urine, stool and skin
- Pregnancy
- Impotence

Antianxiety agents

- Following prescription exactly
- Excessive sedation, unsteadiness (especially in the elderly)
- Other medications used
- Skin rashes
- Pregnancy

In the use of medication in the prolonged management of patients, there is a risk of gradual diminution of thoughtful objectivity in the conduct of the treatment, which may degrade into a routine of occasional superficial "check-ups" and reissuing of prescriptions. This pattern derives from unrealistic and simplistic expectations of chemotherapy, is demoralizing to patients as well as to psychiatrists and their colleagues, and contributes to high drop-out rates and often to the failure of treatment programs. Moreover, such a pattern of indifferent and routine care probably contributes to increased rates of toxic side effects of antipsychotic, antimanic, and antidepressant drugs and to the abuse of antianxiety agents. Furthermore, in a busy clinic or office practice, it is particularly tempting to allow the *"ritualization"* of chemotherapy to displace sensitive and honest attention to painful and difficult psychological and social issues, needs, and wishes of patients. Ritualization of chemotherapy can also encourage patients to overvalue the importance of medications to their continued well-being, and to resist necessary changes of medication. To some extent, such an impasse can be avoided by the encouragement of positive feelings toward the psychiatrist or clinic staff as persons rather than the "magical" pills they provide. Another useful principle is to be prepared to offer something (more time or other psychological support) in place of what the patient feels deprived of and gradually to discontinue a cherished agent.

The management of psychiatric outpatient chemotherapy—a medical treatment—is further complicated by the *sharing of responsibility* for patients and clients among professional and paraprofessional colleagues, many of whom are not medically trained. Treatment by psychiatric teams representing vastly different backgrounds and experience is presently encountered frequently in private as well as public outpatient services. Arrangements for the sharing of clinical responsibilities in outpatient services, as in all forms of psychiatric care, are heavily influenced by forces that are not directly medical or scientific, including the administrative and financial environment. For example, clinical teams representing several disciplines are common in public institutions, hospital clinics, community mental health centers, and some private group practices. Often these arrangements have arisen in part because of the manpower needs and limited funds available for rapidly expanded community mental health services. Economic forces that encourage reliance on clinicians without medical training include support by public funds or grants, rather than private or insured fees. Meeting the requirements of responsible and medically safe care in such a complex environment is not a simple matter.

Treatment with prescription drugs is the medical and legal responsibility of a psychiatrist or other physician on the treatment team, and in this way chemotherapy differs from psychological, social and rehabilitative aspects of work with psychiatric outpatients and clients. Furthermore, a physician is important in the initial evaluation of psychiatric patients, particularly those with psychotic symptoms or other disorders that require consideration of medical conditions in their differential diagnosis and treatment. In addition, a physician is required to prescribe medications, to regulate dosages, to evaluate medically the subsequent responses of the patient, and to manage the treatment when other medical illnesses coexist with the psychiatric conditions. Such activities related to chemotherapy have contributed greatly to the increasingly medical orientation of many general psychiatrists trained since the 1950s.

The administrative mechanisms by which these requirements are met vary considerably with patients' requirements and the personnel and facilities available. When availability of the services of psychiatrists or other physicians is severly limited, their effectiveness can be increased by their serving in a supervisory capacity, in addition to providing an initial examination, and at least brief subsequent direct contacts with the patients. In order to carry out such interdisciplinary outpatient programs, it is increasingly necessary for colleagues without medical training to gain some appreciation for the actions, pharmacology, and toxic effects of drugs used for psychiatric patients, as discussed in this monograph. Thus, a crucial role for the psychiatrist on an outpatient psychiatric treatment team is staff education and, directly or indirectly, patient education as well. In order to achieve adequate medical care in a complex multidisciplinary setting, the effectiveness and safety of chemotherapy and continuing requirements for it are sometimes monitored by the use of explicit and detailed treatment protocols and check lists with which a staff member, other than physician, trained in their use can evaluate a patient on a clinic visit. These typically include behavioral and psychological ratings tailored to the syndrome being treated, along with a record of the medication given, doses, drug blood levels (when available), timing, and the responses of the patient to a specific list of questions as well as the clinician's observations appropriate to the medication in question, and incorporating at least the items listed in Table 22. During each clinic visit in every case, the protocol is evaluated by a psychiatrist or other physician, and appropriate steps are taken before the patient leaves the clinic the same day. A medical evaluation can often be conducted with enhanced benefit to all concerned by inviting the involved staff members to participate in the examination.

Psychological Factors in Chemotherapy

Traditionally psychiatry has been preoccupied with the *process* of psychiatric treatment, and usually that means psychotherapy. This concern has arisen in part from psychoanalytic suggestions that the behavior, utterances and feelings of patients in any setting to some extent reflect typical or characteristic reactions, or even earlier experiences. However, the personal, psychological, and sociological aspects of medical treatments are at least as important as they are to psychotherapy. *Characterological traits* of patients and the nature of their acute *psychological* problems color their way of dealing with medications, and their reactions to chemotherapy and other aspects of their care. Thus, obsessional patients may worry and fuss about details of their treatment and their reactions to it, and may provoke sticky controversies and debates over their treatment. Hysterical or impulsive patients may react to side effects in an exaggerated manner, or abuse medications impulsively. Narcissistic or hypomanic patients are often bothered by any loss of mental or physical capacity perceived as due to a drug, or may refuse to accept the "crutch" of medication at all. Depressed patients may be reluctant to accept medication owing to feelings of hopelessness, worthlessness or anger, and side effects may contribute to their hypochondriacal preoccupations. Schizophrenic patients may cooperate poorly because of suspiciousness, delusions, autistic preoccupation, and perplexity or may become unrealistically dependent on the treatment program and rigidly resistant to changes in it. Sociopathic patients may abuse sedatives, involve a number of clinicians in their abuses, and embroil the clinicians in struggles for control and dominance.

Simplification of Chemotherapy

Chemotherapy can be conducted with greater accuracy, safety, and success by *simplification* of the regimen. Multiple medications are avoided, not only because of the increased risk of complex and sometimes obscure toxicity and drug interactions but also because multiple prescriptions are too difficult to follow faithfully over a long time. Moreover, since antipsychotic agents and antidepressants (in contrast to lithium salts and sedatives) have relatively long half-lives in the body, it is often possible to take an entire day's dose at bedtime, thus simplifying the regimen and at the same time minimizing excessive daytime sedation and autonomic side effects. In addition, for simplicity and savings in cost, the largest available unit of medication (mg per pill) should be prescribed, and small quantities should be dispensed until it is certain that the drug will be used for prolonged periods. At the start of outpatient chemotherapy, it is a good idea to insist that the patient or a family member bring to the clinician *all* bottles of medications of all types that are at home so as to avoid continued use of unnecessary medications, reduce suicidal risks, and avoid potential drug interactions. In addition, a list should be made of all the other physicians involved in the patient's care, and this list and an outline of other coexisting medical treatments should be frequently updated.

Simplification of another type is also important to both inpatient and outpatient psychiatrists. Since many agents in each of the classes discussed in the preceding chapters are more similar than different, and since it is difficult to become clinically and pharmacologically expert on every agent available, it is reasonable to select a small number of agents for inclusion in one's *personal pharmacopoeia*. In making such selections, certain general principles have already been mentioned and can be summarized. Agents should be selected that have been exposed to extensive clinical testing unless there are compelling indications that a new agent has something special to offer. While it is tempting to try every new agent that comes along, if only out of dissatisfaction with older drugs or to make use of novelty for its own sake, the optimistic expectations of new agents in psychopharmacology are usually unrealistic. An important conclusion about the past twenty years of drug development in this field is that there have been remarkably few fundamentally new developments since the 1950s. It is also well to use agents that are readily available in many forms for oral and parenteral use, and to select drugs that are available as generic chemicals, or whose price is known to be competitive locally. A list of drugs used should include at least one representative of the major chemical classes in each division. Thus, among the antipsychotic agents, one aliphatic and one piperidine low-potency phenothiazine might be selected, as well as one or two high-potency phenothiazines, including a depot form, and one butyrophenone. It is important to be aware of the availability of loxitane and molindone if allergic toxic reactions require the use of a chemically unique agent. Lithium need only be used as the generic carbonate salt. Among the antidepressants, only two or three with the best overall results in clinical trials are necessary, and these might include one demethylated agent. Although the MAO inhibitors are not used frequently, one should be familiar with tranylcypromine, and possibly also phenelzine. Among the large sedative-antianxiety group of agents, familiarity with only two or three barbiturates and diphenhydramine among the antihistamines is necessary. Heavy reliance should be placed on not more than three benzodiazepines, including oxazepam and flurazepam, and either diazepam or chlordiazepoxide. To manage neurological side effects of the antipsychotic agents, diphenhydramine can be used for dystonia; diazepam for akathisia; trihexiphenidyl, benztropine, or their equivalent for dystonia, parkinsonism, and akathisia; one should also be familiar with amantadine.

Objectivity in Chemotherapy

The success of psychiatric chemotherapy has led to a class of problems that have been mentioned in previous chapters, but bear repeating. In this book the very term "chemotherapy" has been chosen rather than currently more fashionable alternatives such as "psychopharmacology" to emphasize that these treatments involve the introduction of foreign chemical substances into the body with the hope of modifying the brain, behavior and feelings in beneficial ways. Despite their sometimes impressive successes, these treatments are limited in efficacy, are potentially toxic and expensive, and are not to be undertaken lightly or pursued relentlessly. The general effectiveness and relative simplicity of chemotherapy are highly attractive—so attractive that it is sometimes difficult to know *when to stop* using it. As in any other form of medical or psychiatric treatment, it is important to work constantly toward an honest and objective assessment of the continuing need for a treatment, and of its efficacy, safety, and economy. While such advice sounds almost trivially obvious, its acceptance in practice is painfully difficult.

Many psychiatric conditions are not suitable for medical treatment, or else respond poorly. For example, it is not reasonable to use antipsychotic agents in cases of mild stresses and strains of life, in adolescent turmoil, or characterological disorders. Antianxiety agents are almost never indicated for prolonged use in such conditions although they are legitimately used for brief periods in episodes of acute anxiety. Lithium is another agent currently at high risk for medical misuse, as more and more cases are inappropriately considered to represent manic-depressive illness. Chronic schizophrenia is often helped greatly by antipsychotic agents, but many cases are not convincingly benefited except during periods of acute psychotic turmoil and disorganization, and even those who do seem both to require and to benefit from this form of treatment require regular reevaluations to determine their continuing need for the medication. Antidepressants and stimulants are to be avoided in cases of chronic fatigue or cases of characterological depression, and the only reasonable long-term use of antidepressants at present is in indubitable, severe recurrent unipolar manic-depressive illness.

The other important aspect of excessive zeal in the use of

medications that has already been discussed repeatedly is the use of excessive numbers of medications and unnecessarily high doses. One reason for this problem is the naive use of drugs for theoretical or wishful reasons rather than objectively demonstrated indications with clearly demonstrable, beneficial responses. Examples include treating a "depressed" schizophrenic with an antidepressant, provoking clinical worsening, and then compounding the problem with more antipsychotic drug; giving an antipsychotic agent or more antidepressant to a depressed patient who becomes agitated and mildly delirious with high doses of an antidepressant; using an antiparkinson medication "prophylactically," routinely, and indefinitely with an antipsychotic agent, whether it is needed or not; increasing the dose of an antipsychotic agent in a schizophrenic who is doing poorly, and not changing the treatment even though no further progress is obtained for months; prescribing lithium for indefinite use after an episode of mild neurotic depression, with a history of a similar illness many years previously; adding a barbiturate or flurazepam at bedtime for a schizophrenic patient who receives several doses of chlorpromazine a day; using antipsychotic agents routinely to sedate angry, troublesome, brain-damaged, or retarded, hospitalized or institutionalized patients; using small doses of antipsychotic agents in place of lithium in the prophylactic treatment of affective disorders.

One of the most difficult concepts for many psychiatrists and other psychiatric professionals to grasp is the requirement of thinking about the vicissitudes of their patient's clinical progress *differentially,* and to avoid the temptation to substitute "understanding" for examination, and an interpretation or glib rationalizations for medical appraisal and treatment. This problem is nowhere more common or dangerous than in the use of medications. Many cases of intoxication with antipsychotic agents, lithium, antidepressants, or sedatives could be avoided or minimized if *early changes* in the *mental status* as evaluated in even a superficial medical examination were recognized as organic, although superimposed upon functional mental illnesses. In this situation, a common error is to recognize clinical worsening, but to assume that worsening must be an exacerbation of the primary diagnosis. The mistreatment that follows often includes inappropriate increases of the dose of one drug, or the addition of other toxic agents to complicate matters further. The best protection against this kind of trap is to maintain a high index of suspicion about toxic responses to medication, and then to *stop the treatment if there is any doubt* about the diagnosis. There is little chance that being proven wrong in this decision will be as dangerous as persisting in, or increasing, a toxic treatment.

Summary

Some of the special problems associated with the use of psychotropic agents in children and elderly patients, and the management of outpatients were emphasized in this chapter. Pediatric and geriatric psychopharmacology are relatively underdeveloped fields. The categorization of behavioral disorders in children and resistance to experimentation with children have limited the development of pediatric psychopharmacology. The elderly are at increased risk of toxic effects of all chemotherapeutic agents. Physiological resilience and metabolic resistance to drugs diminish with advancing age and often result in behavioral or other manifestations of drug intoxication at doses readily tolerated by younger patients. The effectiveness and safety of chemotherapy can be greatly enhanced by attention to the psychological and social aspects of the individuals involved and the setting in which the treatment is carried out. Simplification and an objective evaluation of the need for chemotherapy and the responses to it greatly increase the efficiency and safety of this form of treatment of psychiatric patients.

BIBLIOGRAPHY / INDEX

Bibliography

General Reviews and Monographs

Appleton, W. S. Third psychoactive drug usage guide *Dis. Nerv. Syst.* 37:39–51, 1976.

Appleton, W. S., and Davis, J. M. *Practical Clinical Psychopharmacology.* Medcom, New York, 1973.

Ayd, F. J., and Blackwell, B., eds. *Discoveries in Biological Psychiatry.* Lippincott, Philadelphia, 1970.

Ayd. F. J. *Rational Psychopharmacotherapy and the Right to Treatment.* Ayd Medical Communications, Baltimore, 1974.

Ban, T. A. *Psychopharmacology.* Williams and Wilkins, Baltimore, 1969.

Ban, T. A. Clinical Pharmacology and Psychiatry. *Dis Nerv. Syst.* 36:612–616, 1975.

Bente, D., and Bradley, P., eds. *Neuropharmacology.* Elsevier, Amsterdam, 1965.

Caffey, E. M., Kaim, S. C., Hollister, L. E., and Pokorny, A. D. *Drug Treatment in Psychiatry.* Veterans Administration, Washington, D. C., 1970.

Clark, W. G., and Del Guidice, J., eds. *Principles of Psychopharmacology.* Academic Press, New York, 1970.

Cole, J. O., and Davis, J. M. Antipsychotic drugs. In *The Schizophrenic Syndrome,* Bellak, L., and Loeb, L., eds. Grune and Stratton, New York, 1969.

Detre, T. P. and Jarecki, H. G. *Modern Psychiatric Treatment.* Lippincott, Philadelphia, 1971.

DiMascio, A., and Shader, R. I. *Clinical Handbook of Psychopharmacology*. Science House, New York, 1970.

Efron, D. H., ed. *Psychopharmacology: A Review of Progress, 1957–1967*, U. S. Public Health Service Publication No. 1836. U. S. Government Printing Office, Washington, D. C., 1968.

Eisenberg, L., and Conners, C. K. Psychopharmacology in childhood. In *Behavioral Science in Pediatric Medicine*, Talbot, N. B., Kagan, J.; and Eisenberg, L., eds. Saunders, Philadelphia, 1971.

Gittelman, R. K., Klein, D. F., and Pollack, M. Effects of Psychotropic drugs on long-term adjustment: a review. *Psychopharmacologia* 5:317–338, 1964.

Gordon, M., ed. *Psychopharmacological Agents*. Academic Press, New York, 1964.

Hollister, L. E. *Clinical Use of Psychotherapeutic Drugs*. Charles C Thomas, Springfield, Ill., 1973.

Hollister, L. E. Drugs for emotional disorders. *J. A. M. A.* 234:942–947, 1975.

Irwin, S. How to prescribe psychoactive drugs. The uses and relative hazard potential of psychoactive drugs. *Bull. Menninger Clin.* 38:1–48, 1974.

Kalinowsky, L. B., and Hippius, H. *Pharmacological, Convulsive and Other Somatic Treatments in Psychiatry*. Grune and Stratton, New York, 1969.

Klein D. F. Importance of psychiatric diagnosis in prediction of clinical drug effects. *Arch. Gen. Psychiatry* 16:18–26, 1967.

Klein, D. F. *Psychiatric Case Studies: Treatment, Drugs and Outcome*. Williams and Wilkins, Baltimore, 1972.

Klein, D. F., and Davis, J. M. *Diagnosis and Drug Treatment of Psychiatric Disorders*. Williams and Wilkins, Baltimore, 1969.

Levitt, R. A., ed. *Psychopharmacology, A Biological Approach*. John Wiley, New York, 1975.

Marks, J., and Pare, C., eds. *The Scientific Basis of Drug Therapy in Psychiatry*. Pergamon Press, New York, 1965.

Phillis, J. W. *The Pharmacology of Synapses*. Pergamon Press, Oxford, 1970.

Rech, R. H., and Moore, K. E., eds. *An Introduction to Psychopharmacology*. Raven Press, New York, 1971.

Shader, R. I., ed. *Manual of Psychiatric Therapeutics. Practical Psychopharmacology and Psychiatry*. Little, Brown, Boston, 1975

Solomon, P., *Psychiatric Drugs*. Grune and Stratton, New York, 1966.

Usdin, E., and Efron, D. E., eds. *Psychotropic Drugs and Related Compounds*, U. S. Public Health Service Publication No. 1589. U. S. Government Printing Office, Washington, D. C., 1967.

Valzelli, L. *Psychopharmacology: An Introduction to Experimental and Clinical Principles*. Spectrum, Flushing, N. Y., 1973.

General Aspects of Psychopharmacology

Altman, H., Mehta, D., Evensen, R., and Sletten, I. W. Behavioral effects of drug therapy on psychogeriatric in-patients. *J. Am. Geriatr. Soc.* 21:241–252, 1973.

Appleton, W. S. Legal problems in psychiatric drug prescription. *Am. J. Psychiatry* 124:877–882, 1968.

Baldessarini, R. J. Frequency of diagnosis of schizophrenia vs. affective disorders from 1944–1968. *Am. J. Psychiatry* 127:759–763, 1970.

Baldessarini, R. J. Biogenic amine hypotheses in affective disorders. In *The Nature and Treatment of Depression*, Flach, F. F., and Draghi, S. C., eds. John Wiley, New York, 1975, pp. 347–385.

Bender, A. D. Pharmacodynamic principles of drug therapy in the aged. *J. Am. Geriatr. Soc.* 22:296–303, 1974.

Bok, S. The ethics of giving placebos. *Sci. Am.* 231:17–23, 1974.

Blackwell, B. Patient compliance with drug therapy. *N. Engl. J. Med.* 289:249–252, 1973.

Cronnie, B. W. The feet of clay of the double-blind trial. *Lancet* 2:994–997, 1963.

Davis, J. M. Psychopharmacology in the aged: Use of psychotropic drugs in geriatric patients. *J. Geriatr. Psychiatry* 7:145–159, 1974.

Dawson-Butterworth, K. The chemotherapeutics of geriatric sedation. *J. Am. Geriatr. Soc.* 18:97–114, 1970.

DeFelice, S. An analysis of the relationship between human experimentation and drug discovery in the United States. *Drug Metab. Rev.* 3:167–184, 1974.

Eisdorfer, C., and Fann, W. E., eds. *Psychopharmacology and Aging*. Plenum, New York, 1973.

Eveloff, H. H. Pediatric psychopharmacology. In *Principles of Psy-*

chopharmacology. Clark, W. G., and Del Guidice, J., eds., Academic Press, New York, 1970, pp. 683–694.

Fish, B. Drug use in psychiatric disorders of children. *Am. J. Psychiatry* 124(Suppl.):31–36, 1968.

Hammar, C. G., Holmstedt, B., Lindgren, J. E., and Thom, R. The combination of gas chromatography and mass spectrometry in the identification of drugs and metabolites. *Adv. Pharmacol. Chemother.* 7:53–65, 1969.

Kastenbaum, R., Slater, P. E., and Aisenberg, R. Toward a conceptual model of geriatric psychopharmacology: an experiment with thioridazine and dextroamphetamine. *Gerontologist* 4:68–71, 1964.

Lasagna, L., Mosteller, F., Felsinger, J., and Bucher, H. A study of the placebo response. *Am. J. Med.* 16:770–779, 1954.

Learoyd, B. M. Psychotropic drugs and the elderly patient. *Med. J. Aust.* 1:1131–1133, 1972.

Lipman, R. S. Pharmacotherapy of children (bibliography). *Psychopharmacol. Bull.* 7:14–30, 1971.

Merlis, S., Sheppard, C., Collins, L., and Fiorentino, D. Polypharmacy in psychiatry: patterns of differential treatment. *Am. J. Psychiatry* 126:1647–1651, 1970.

Muller, C. The overmedicated society: Forces in the marketplace for medical care. *Science* 176:488–492, 1972.

Plutchik, R., Platman, S. and Fieve, R. Three alternatives to the double-blind. *Arch. Gen. Psychiatry* 20:428–432, 1950.

Park, L. C., and Imboden, J. B. Chemical and heuristic value of clinical drug research. *J. Nerv. Ment. Dis.* 151:322–340, 1970.

Prien, R. F., Haber, P. A., and Caffey, E. M. The use of psychoactive drugs in elderly patients with psychiatric disorders: survey conducted in twelve Veterans Administration hospitals. *J. Am. Geriatr. Soc.* 23:104–112, 1975.

Quay, H. C., and Werry, J. S., eds. *Psychopathological Disorders of Childhood.* John Wiley, New York, 1972.

Rickels, K. *Non-specific Factors in Drug Therapy.* Charles C Thomas, Springfield, Ill., 1968.

Rosenthal, R. Experimenter outcome-orientation and the results of the psychological experiment. *Psychol. Bull.* 61:405–412, 1964.

Ross, S., Krugman, A., Lyerly, S., and Clyde, D. Drugs and placebos: a model design. *Psychol. Rep.* 10:383–392, 1962.

Schildkraut, J. J. *Neuropsychopharmacology and the Affective Disorders.* Little, Brown, Boston, 1970.

Spencer, P. S. J. Animal models for screening new agents. *Br. J. Clin. Pharmacol.* (Suppl.):5–12, 1976.

Sprague, R. L., and Werry, J. S. Pediatric psychopharmacology. *Psychopharmacol. Bull.* (Special issue, *Pharmacotherapy of Children*):21–23, 1973.

Sudilovsky, A., Gershon, S., and Beer, B., eds. *Predictability in Psychopharmacology: Preclinical and Clinical Correlations.* Raven Press, New York, 1975.

Wittenborn, J. R., and May, P. R., eds. *Prediction of Response to Pharmacotherapy.* Charles C Thomas, Springfield, Ill., 1966.

Wolf, S. The pharmacology of placebos. *Pharmacol. Rev.* 11:689–704, 1959.

Antipsychotic Chemicals

Alpert, M., Diamond, F., and Laski, E. M. Anticholinergic exacerbation of phenothiazine-induced extrapyramidal syndrome. *Am. J. Psychiatry* 133:1073–1075, 1976.

Alvarez-Mena, S. C., and Frank, M. J. Phenothiazine-induced T-wave abnormalities. *J. A. M. A.* 224:1730–1733, 1973.

American Psychiatric Association Task Force (Lipton, M. A., Chairman). *Megavitamin and Orthomolecular Therapy in Psychiatry,* Task Force Report No. 7. American Psychiatric Association, Washington, D. C., 1973.

Anderson, W. H., and Kuehnle, J. C. Strategies for the treatment of acute psychosis. *J. A. M. A.* 229:1884–1889, 1974.

Anderson, W. H., Kuehnle, J. C., and Catanzano, D. M. Rapid treatment of psychosis. *Am. J. Psychiatry* 133:1076–1078, 1976.

Ayd, F. J. Cardiovascular effects of phenothiazines. *Int. Drug Ther. Newsletter* 5:1–8, 1970.

Ayd, F. J. Rational pharmacotherapy: once-a-day drug dosage. *Dis. Nerv. Syst.* 34:371–373, 1973.

Ban, T. A. Haloperidol and the butyrophenones. *Psychosomatics* 14:286–297, 1973.

Barton, R., and Hurst, L. Unnecessary use of tranquilizers in elderly patients. *Brit. J. Psychiatry* 112:989–990, 1966.

Beumont, P. J. V., Corker, C. S., Friesen, H. G., et al. The effects of phenothiazines on endocrine function. II. Effect in men and post-menopausal women. *Brit. J. Psychiatry* 124:420–430, 1974.

Beumont, P. J. V., Gelder, M. G., Friesen, H. G., et al. The effects of phenothiazines on endocrine function. I. Patients with inappropriate lactation and amenorrhoea. *Brit. J. Psychiatry* 124:413–419, 1974.

Bowers, M. B., Jr., and Rozitis, A. Regional differences in homovanillic acid concentrations after acute and chronic administration of antipsychotic drugs. *J. Pharm. Pharmacol.* 26:743–745, 1974.

Bunney, B. S., Walters, J. R., Roth, R. H., and Aghajanian, G. K. Dopaminergic neurons: effect of antipsychotic drugs and amphetamine on single cell activity. *J. Pharmacol. Exp. Ther.* 185:560–571, 1973.

Burgoyne, R. W. Effect of drug ritual change on schizophrenic patients. *Am. J. Psychiatry* 133:284–289, 1976.

Bürki, A. R., Ruch, W., and Asper, H. Effects of clozapine, thioridazine, perlapine and haloperidol on the metabolism of the biogenic amines in the brain of the rat. *Psychopharmacologia* 41:27–33, 1975.

Burt, D. R., Enna, S. J., Creese, I., and Snyder, S. H. Dopamine receptor binding in the corpus striatum of mammalian brain. *Proc. Natl. Acad. Sci. USA* 72:4655–4659, 1975.

Caffey, E. M., Diamond, L., Frank, T., et al. Discontinuation or reduction of chemotherapy in chronic schizophrenics. *J. Chronic Dis.* 17:347–358, 1964.

Campbell, M. Biological interventions in psychoses of childhood. *J. Autism Child. Schizo.* 3:347–373, 1973.

Callahan, E. J., Alevizos, P. N., Teigen, J. R., et al. Behavioral effects of reducing the daily frequency of phenothiazine administration. *Arch. Gen. Psychiatry* 32:1285–1290, 1975.

Casey, J. F., Lasky, J., Klett, C., and Hollister, L. Treatment of schizophrenic reactions with phenothiazine derivatives: a comparative study. *Am. J. Psychiatry* 117:97–105, 1960.

Chapman, L. J., and Knowles, R. R. The effects of phenothiazine on disordered thought in schizophrenia. *J. Consult. Psychol.* 28:165–169, 1964.

Chien, C. P., DiMascio, A., and Cole, J. O. Antiparkinson agents and depot phenothiazine. *Am. J. Psychiatry* 131:86–90, 1974.

Chouinard, G., Pinard, G., Prenoveau, Y., and Tetreault, L. Potentiation of haloperidol by alpha-methyltyrosine in the treatment of schizophrenic patients. *Curr. Ther. Res.* 15:473–483, 1973.

Cole, J. O. Phenothiazine treatment in acute schizophrenia. *Arch. Gen. Psychiatry* 10:246–261, 1964.

Cole, J. O., ed. Symposium on long-acting phenothiazines in psychiatry. *Dis. Nerv. Syst.* 31(Suppl.):1–71, 1970.

Cohen, M. M., Hirschhorn, K., and Frosch, W. A. Cytogenetic effects of tranquilizing drugs in vivo and in vitro. *J. A. M. A.* 207:2425–2426, 1969.

Costall, B., and Naylor, R. J. Mesolimbic involvement with behavioral effects indicating antipsychotic activity. *Eur. J. Pharmacol.* 27:46–58, 1974.

Courvoisier, S., Fournel, J., Ducrot, R., et al. Properties pharmacodynamiques du chlorhydrate de chloro-3-(dimethyl-amino-3'-propyl)-10-phenothiazine (4560 RP). *Arch. Int. Pharmacodyn. Ther.* 92:305–361, 1952.

Crane, G. E. A review of clinical literature on haloperidol. *Int. J. Neuropsychiatry* 3(Suppl.):110–123, 1967.

Creese, I., Burt, D. R., and Snyder, S. H. Dopamine receptor binding predicts clinical and pharmacological potencies of antischizophrenic drugs. *Science* 192:481–483, 1976.

Curry, S. H., Marshall, J. H. L., Davis, J. M., and Janowsky, D. S. Chlorpromazine plasma levels and effects. *Arch. Gen. Psychiatry* 22:289–296, 1970.

Davidorf, F. H. Thioridazine pigmentary retinopathy. *Arch. Ophthalmol.* 90:251–255, 1973.

Davis, J. M. Comparative doses and costs of antipsychotic medication. *Arch. Gen. Psychiatry* 33:858–861, 1976.

Davis, J. M. Overview: Maintenance therapy in psychiatry. I. Schizophrenia. *Am. J. Psychiatry* 132:1237–1245, 1975.

Davis, J. M. Recent developments in the treatment of schizophrenia. *Psychiatr. Annals* 6:71–111, 1976.

Davis, J. M., and Cole, J. O. Antipsychotic drugs. *Comprehensive Textbook of Psychiatry II.* Freedman, A. M., Kaplan, H. I., and Sadock, B. J., eds. Williams and Wilkins, Baltimore, 1975, pp. 1921–1941.

Delay, J., Deniker, P., and Harl, J. Utilization therapeutique psychiatrique d'une phenothiazine d'action centrale elective (4560 RP). *Ann. med. Psychol.* 110:112–117, 1952.

Denber, H., and Bird, E. Chlorpromazine in the treatment of mental illness IV. Final results with analysis of data on 1,523 patients. *Am. J. Psychiatry* 113:972–978, 1957.

Dimond, R. C., Brammer, S. R., Atkinson, R. L., Jr., et al. Chlorpromazine treatment and growth hormone secretory responses in acromegaly. *J. Clin. Endocrinol. Metab.* 36:1189–1195, 1973.

Donlon, P. T., and Tupin, J. P. Rapid "digitalization" of decompensated schizophrenic patients with antipsychotic agents. *Am. J. Psychiatry* 131:310–312, 1974.

Engelhardt, D. M., Polizos, P., Waizer, J., and Hoffman, S. P. A double-blind comparison of fluphenazine and haloperidol. *J. Autism Child. Schizo.* 3:128–137, 1973.

Engelhardt, D. M., Rosen, B., Freedman, N., and Margolis, R. Phenothiazines in prevention of psychiatric hospitalization—a reevaluation. *Arch. Gen. Psychiatry* 16:98–101, 1967.

Ericksen, S. E., Hurt, S. W., and Davis, J. M. Dosage of antipsychotic drugs. *N. Engl. J. Med.* 294:1296–1297, 1976.

Faretra, G., Dooher, L., and Dowling, J. Comparisons of haloperidol and fluphenazine in disturbed children. *Am. J. Psychiatry* 126:1670–1673, 1970.

Feinberg, A. P., and Snyder, S. H. Phenothiazine drugs: structure-activity relationships explained by a conformation mimics dopamine. *Proc. Natl. Acad. Sci. USA* 72:1899–1903, 1975.

Fletcher, G. F., and Wenger, N. K. Cardiotoxic effects of Mellaril: conduction disturbances and supraventricular arrhythmias. *Am. Heart J.* 78:135–138, 1969.

Forrest, I. S., Bolt, A. G., and Serra, M. T. Distribution of chlorpromazine metabolites in selected organs of psychiatric patients chronically dosed up to the time of death. *Biochem. Pharmacol.* 17:2061–2070, 1968.

Forrest, I. S., Carr, C. J., and Usdin, E., eds. *Phenothiazines and Structurally Related Drugs*. Raven Press, New York, 1974.

Galbrecht, C. R., and Klett, C. J. Predicting response to phenothiazines: The right drug for the right patient. *J. Nerv. Ment. Dis.* 147:173–183, 1968.

Gardos, G., and Cole, J. O. The dual action of thiothixene. *Arch. Gen. Psychiatry* 29:222–225, 1973.

Gardos, G., and Cole, J. O. Maintenance antipsychotic therapy: is the cure worse than the disease? *Am. J. Psychiatry* 133:32–36, 1976.

Garver, D. L., Davis, J. M., Dekirmenjian, H., et al. Pharmacokinetics of red blood cell phenothiazine and clinical effects. *Arch. Gen. Psychiatry* 33:862–866, 1976.

Gelenberg, A. J., and Mandel, M. R. Catatonic reactions to high potency neuroleptic drugs. *Arch. Gen. Psychiatry (In press)*.

Goldberg, S. C., Frosch, W. A., Drossman, A. K., et al. Prediction of response to phenothiazines in schizophrenia: A cross validation study. *Arch. Gen. Psychiatry* 26:367–373, 1972.

Grabowski, S. W. Safety and effectiveness of haloperidol for mentally retarded behaviorally disordered and hyperkinetic patients. *Curr. Ther. Res.* 15:856–861, 1973.

Gram, L. F., and Rafaelsen, O. J. Lithium treatment of psychotic children and adolescents: a controlled clinical trial. *Acta Psychiatr. Scand.* 48:253–260, 1972.

Greenblatt, M., Solomon, M. H., Evans, A. S., and Brooks, G. W., eds. *Drug and Social Therapy in Schizophrenia*. Charles C Thomas, Springfield, Ill., 1965.

Greiner, A., and Berry, K. Skin pigmentation and corneal and lens opacities with prolonged chlorpromazine therapy. *Canad. Med. Assoc, J.* 90:663–665, 1964.

Grinspoon, L., Ewalt, J. R., and Shader, R. I. *Schizophrenia: Pharmacotherapy and Psychotherapy*. Williams and Wilkins, Baltimore, 1972.

Grinspoon, L., Ewalt, J. R., and Shader, R. Psychotherapy and pharmacotherapy in chronic schizophrenia. *Am. J. Psychiatry* 124:1645–1652, 1968.

Groves, J. E., and Mandel, M. R. The long-acting phenothiazines. *Arch. Gen. Psychiatry* 32:893–900, 1975.

Groves, P. M., and Rebec, G. V. Biochemistry and behavior: some central actions of amphetamine and antipsychotic drugs. *Ann. Rev. Psychol.* 27:91–127, 1976.

Hanlon, T. E., Michaux, M., Ota, K., et al. The comparative effectiveness of 8 phenothiazines. *Psychopharmacologia* 7:89–106, 1965.

Hogarty, G. E., Goldberg, S. C., and The Collaborative Study Group: Drugs and sociotherapy in the aftercare of schizophrenic patients. One-year relapse rates. *Arch. Gen. Psychiatry* 28:54–62, 1973.

Hollister, L. E., Curry, S. H., Derr, J. E., and Kanter, S. L. Studies of delayed action medication. V. Plasma levels and urinary excretion of chlorpromazine in four different dosage forms given acutely and in steady state conditions. *Clin. Pharmacol. Ther.* 11:49–59, 1970.

Hollister, L. E., Overall, J. E., Kimbell, I., and Pokorny, A. Specific indications for different classes of phenothiazines. *Arch. Gen. Psychiatry* 30:94–99, 1974.

Honigfeld, G., Rosenblum, M. P., Blumenthal, I. J., et al. Behavioral improvement in the older schizophrenic patient: drug and social therapies. *J. Am. Geriatr. Soc.* 13:57–71, 1965.

Hordern, A. Psychiatry and the tranquilizers. *N. Engl. J. Med.* 265:584–634, 1961.

Iversen, L. L. Dopamine receptors in the brain. *Science* 188:1084–1089, 1975.

Jacobson, G., Baldessarini, R. J., and Manschreck, T. Tardive and withdrawal dyskinesia associated with haloperidol. *Am. J. Psychiatry* 131:910–913, 1974.

Janssen, P. A. J. Chemical and pharmacological classification of neuroleptics. In *Modern Problems in Pharmacopsychiatry: The Neuroleptics,* Bokon, O. P., Janssen, P. A. J., and Bokon, J., eds., Vol. 5. S. Karger, Basel, 1970, pp. 34–44.

Janssen, P. A. J. Long-acting neuroleptics and other psychoactive drugs of the future. *Clin. Med.* 79:12–14, 1972.

Janssen, P. A. J., Niemegeers, C. J. E., and Schellekens, K. H. L. Is it possible to predict the clinical effects of neuroleptics drugs (major tranquilizers) from animal data? II. Neuroleptic activity spectra for drugs. *Arzneim. Forsch.* 15:1196–1206, 1965.

Kiev, A. Double-blind comparison of thiothixene and protriptyline in psychotic depression. *Dis. Nerv. Syst.* 33:811–816, 1973.

Kirven, L. E., and Montero, E. F. Comparison of thioridazine and diazepam on the control of nonpsychiatric symptoms associated with senility: double blind study. *J. Am. Geriatr. Soc.* 21:546–551, 1973.

Klawans, H. L., Jr., Bergen, D., and Bruyn, G. W. Prolonged drug-induced parkinsonism. *Confin. Neurol.* 35:368–377, 1973.

Klawans, H. L., Jr., Bergen, D., Bruyn, G. W., and Paulson, G. W. Neuroleptic-induced tardive dyskinesias in nonpsychotic patients. *Arch. Neurol.* 30:338–339, 1974.

Klett, C. J., and Caffey, E. M., Jr. Evaluating the long-term need for antiparkinson drugs by chronic schizophrenics. *Arch. Gen. Psychiatry* 26:374–379, 1972.

Kopelman, A. E., McCullar, F. W., and Heggeness, L. Limb malformations following maternal use of haloperidol. *J. A. M. A.* 231:62–64, 1975.

Korein, J., Fish, B., Shapiro, T., et al. EEG and behavior effects on drug therapy in children: chlorpromazine and diphenhydramine. *Arch. Gen. Psychiatry* 24:552–563, 1971.

Lasky, J. J., Klett, C. J., Caffey, E. M., Jr., et al. Drug treatment of schizophrenic patients: A comparative evaluation of chlorpromazine, chlorprothixene, fluphenazine, reserpine, thioridazine and triflupromazine, *Dis. Nerv. Syst.* 23:298–306, 1962.

Leemsta, J. E., and Koenig, K. L. Sudden death and phenothiazines. A current controversy. *Arch. Gen. Psychiatry* 18:137–148, 1968.

Lee, P. A., Kelly, M. R., and Wallin, J. D. Increased prolactin levels during reserpine treatment of hypertensive patients. *J. A. M. A.* 235:2316–2317, 1976.

Lehmann, H. F., Ban, T. A., and Suxena, B. M. Nicotinic acid, thioridazine, fluoxymesterone and their combinations in hospitalized geriatric patients. *Am. Psychiatr. Soc. J.* 17:315–320, 1972.

Lehmann, H. E., and Hanrahan, G. E. Chlorpromazine, a new inhibiting agent for psychomotor excitement and manic states. *A. M. A. Arch. Neurol. Psychiatry* 71:227–237, 1954.

Lord, D. J., and Kidd, C. B. Haloperidol versus diazepam: A double-blind crossover clinical trial. *Med. J. Austr.* 1:586–588, 1973.

McAndrew, J. B., Case, Q., and Treffert, D. Effects of prolonged phenothiazine intake on psychotic and other hospitalized children. *J. Autism Child. Schizo.* 2:75–91, 1972.

McClelland, H. A., Blessed, G., Bhate, S., Ali, N., and Clarke, P. A. The abrupt withdrawal of antiparkinsonian drugs in schizophrenic patients. *Brit. J. Psychiatry* 124:151–159, 1974.

Man, P. L., and Chen, C. H. Rapid tranquilization of acutely psychotic patients with intramuscular haloperidol and chlorpromazine. *Psychosomatics* 14:59–63, 1973.

Marks, J. Pre-drug behavior as a predictor of response to phenothiazines among schizophrenics. *J. Nerv. Ment. Dis.* 137:597–601, 1963.

Mason, A. S. Basic principles in the use of antipsychotic agents. *Hosp. Community Psychiatry* 24:825–829, 1973.

Matthysse, S. Antipsychotic drug actions: a clue to the neuropathology of schizophrenia? *Fed. Proc.* 32:200–205, 1973.

May, P. R. A. Rational treatment for an irrational disorder: What does the schizophrenic patient need? *Am. J. Psychiatry* 133:1008–1012, 1976.

May, P. R. A. *Treatment of Schizophrenia: A Comparative Study of Five Treatment Methods.* Science House, New York, 1968.

Messiha, F. S., Knopp, W., Vanecko, S., et al. Haloperidol therapy in Tourette's syndrome: neurophysiological, biochemical and behavioral correlates. *Life Sci.* 10:449–457, 1971.

Miller, R. J., Horn, A. S., and Iversen, L. L. The action of neuroleptic drugs on dopamine-stimulated adenosine cyclic 3′,5′-monophosphate production in rat neostriatum and limbic forebrain. *Mol. Pharmacol.* 10:759–766, 1974.

Møller-Nielsen, I., Pedersen, V., Nymark, M., et al. The comparative pharmacology of flupenthixol and some reference neuroleptics. *Acta Pharmacol. Toxicol.* (Kbh.) 33:353–362, 1973.

Mones, R. J. The use of haloperidol in neurologic patients. In *Butyrophenones in Psychiatry,* DiMascio, A., and Shader, R. I., eds. Raven Press, New York, 1972.

Mosher, L. R. Nicotinic acid side-effects and toxicity: A review. *Am. J. Psychiatry* 126:1290–1296, 1970.

Nasrallah, H. A., Donnelly, E. F., Bigelow, L. B., et al. Effects of alpha-methyl-para-tyrosine on medicated chronic schizophrenics. *Arch. Gen. Psychiatry* (in press).

National Institute of Mental Health Psychopharmacology Service Center Collaborative Study Group. Phenothiazine treatment in acute schizophrenia. *Arch. Gen. Psychiatry* 10:246–261, 1964.

Oldham, A. J., and Bott, M. The management of excitement in a general hospital psychiatric ward by high dosage haloperidol. *Acta Psychiatr. Scand.* 47:369–376, 1971.

Orlov, P., Kasparian, G., DiMascio, A., and Cole, J. O. Withdrawal of antiparkinson drugs. *Arch. Gen. Psychiatry* 25:246–261, 1964.

Petersen, P. V., and Møller-Nielsen, I. Thioxanthene derivatives. In *Psychopharmacological Agents,* Gordon, M., ed., Vol. 1. Academic Press, New York, 1964.

Pisciotta, A. V. Agranulocytosis induced by certain phenothiazine derivatives. *J. A. M. A.* 208:1862–1868, 1969.

Polizos, P., Engelhardt, D. M., Hoffman, S. P., and Waizer, J. Neurological consequences of psychotropic drug withdrawal in schizophrenic children. *J. Autism Child. Schizo.* 3:247–253, 1973.

Post, R. M., and Goodwin, F. K. Time-dependent effects of phenothiazines on dopamine turnover in psychiatric patients. *Science* 190:488–489, 1975.

Prien, R. F., Cole, J. O., and Belkin, N. F. Relapse in chronic schizophrenics following abrupt withdrawal of tranquilizing medication. *Brit. J. Psychiatry* 115:679–686, 1969.

Prien, R. F., DeLong, S. L., Cole, J. O., and Levine, J. Ocular changes occurring with prolonged high dose chlorpromazine therapy. *Arch. Gen. Psychiatry* 23:464–468, 1970.

Pritchard, M. Prognosis of schizophrenia before and after pharmacotherapy. II. Three-year follow up. *Brit. J. Psychiatry* 113:1353–1359, 1967.

Quitkin, F., Rifkin, A., and Klein, D. F. Very high dosage vs. standard dosage fluphenazine in schizophrenia. *Arch. Gen. Psychiatry* 32:1276–1281, 1975.

Rivera-Calimlim, L., Casteneda, L., and Lasagna, L. Effects of mode of management on plasma chlorpromazine in psychiatric patients. *Clin. Pharmacol. Ther.* 14:978–986, 1973.

Rivera-Calimlim, L., Nasrallah, H., Strauss, J., and Lasagna, L. Clinical response and plasma levels: Effect of dose, dosage schedules, and drug interactions on plasma chlorpromazine levels. *Am. J. Psychiatry* 133:646–652, 1976.

Seeman, P. The membrane actions of anesthetics and tranquilizers. *Pharmacol. Rev.* 24:583–655, 1972.

Seeman, P., Chau-Wong, M., Tedesco, J., and Wong, K. Brain receptors for antipsychotic drugs and dopamine: direct binding assays. *Proc. Natl. Acad. Sci. USA* 72:4376–4380, 1975.

Seeman, P., Lee, T., Chau-Wong, M., and Wong, K. Antipsychotic drug doses and neuroleptic/dopamine receptors. *Nature* 261:717–719, 1976.

Sen, G., and Bose, K. C. *Rauwolfia serpentina,* a new Indian drug for insanity and high blood pressure. *Ind. Med. World* 2:194–201, 1931.

Serrano, A. C., and Forbis, O. L. Haloperidol for psychiatric disorders in children. *Dis. Nerv. Syst.* 34:226–231, 1973.

Shapiro, A. K., Shapiro, E., and Wayne, H. Treatment of Tourette's syndrome. *Arch. Gen. Psychiatry* 28:92–97, 1973.

Shopsin, B., Kim, S. S., and Gershon, S. A controlled study of lithium vs. chlorpromazine in acute schizophrenics. *Brit. J. Psychiatry* 119:435–440, 1971.

Simpson, G. M., and Varga, E. Clozapine—a new antipsychotic agent. *Curr. Ther. Res.* 16:679–686, 1974.

Singh, M. M., and Kay, S. R. A comparative study of haloperidol and chlorpromazine in terms of clinical effects and therapeutic reversal with benztropine in schizophrenia. *Psychopharmacologia* 43:103–113, 1975.

Smith, K., Surphlis, W., Gynter, M., and Shimkunas, A. ECT and chlorpromazine compared in the treatment of schizophrenia. *J. Nev. Ment. Dis.* 144:284–290, 1967.

Snyder, S., Greenberg, D., and Yamamura, H. I. Antischizophrenic drugs and brain cholinergic receptors. *Arch. Gen. Psychiatry* 31:58–61, 1974.

Snyder, S. H., Taylor, K. M., Coyle, J. T., and Meyerhoff, J. L. The role of brain dopamine in behavioral regulation and the actions of psychotropic drugs. *Am. J. Psychiatry* 127:199–207, 1970.

Stawarz, R. J., Hill, H., Robinson, S. E., et al. On the significance of the increase in homovanillic acid (HVA) caused by antipsychotic drugs in corpus striatum and limbic forebrain. *Psychopharcologia* 43:125–130, 1975.

Swazey, J. *Chlorpromazine: The History of the Psychiatric Discovery.* M. I. T. Press, Cambridge, Mass., 1974.

Tarsy, D., and Baldessarini, R. J. The tardive dyskinesia syndrome. In *Clinical Neuropharmacology,* Klawans, H., ed., Raven Press, New York, 1976, pp. 29–61.

Tobias, L. L., and MacDonald, M. L. Withdrawal of maintenance drugs with long-term hospitalized mental patients. *Psychol. Bull.* 81:107–125, 1974.

Tsuang, M. M., Lu, L. M., Stotsky, B. A., and Cole, J. O. Haloperidol vs. thioridazine for hospitalized psychogeriatric patients: double-blind study. *J. Am. Geriatr. Soc.* 19:593–600, 1971.

VanPutten, T. Why do schizophrenic patients refuse to take their drugs? *Arch. Gen. Psychiatry* 31:67–72, 1974.

Waizer, J., Polizos, P., Hoffman, S. P., et al. A single-blind evaluation of thiothixene with out-patient schizophrenic children. *J. Autism Child. Schizo.* 2:378–386, 1972.

Warner, A. M., and Wyman, S. M. Delayed severe extrapyramidal disturbance following frequent depot phenothiazine administration. *Am. J. Psychiatry* 132:743–745, 1975.

Weissman, A. Chemical, pharmacological, and metabolic considerations on thiothixene. In *Thiothixene and the Thioxanthenes,*

Forrest, I. S., Carr, C. J., and Usdin, E., eds. Raven Press, New York, 1974, pp. 1–10.

Werry, J. S., Weiss, G., Douglas, V., and Martin, J. Studies on the hyperactive child. III. The effect of chlorpromazine upon behavior and learning ability. *J. Am. Acad. Child. Psychiatry* 5:292–312, 1966.

Wijsenbeek, H., Steiner, M., and Goldberg, S. C. Trifluoperazine: a comparison between regular and high doses. *Psychopharmacologia* 36:147–150, 1974.

Lithium Salts

Agulnik, P. L., DiMascio, A., and Moore, P. Acute brain syndrome associated with lithium therapy. *Am. J. Psychiatry* 129:621–623, 1972.

Baastrup, P. C., Paulsen, J. C., Schou, M., and Thomsen, K. Prophylactic lithium: double-blind discontinuation in manic-depressive and recurrent depressive disorders. *Lancet* 2:326–330, 1970.

Baldessarini, R. J., and Lipinski, J. F. Lithium salts: 1970–1975. *Ann. Intern. Med.* 83:527–533, 1975.

Baldessarini, R. J., and Stephens, J. H. Lithium carbonate for affective disorders. I. Clinical pharmacology and toxicology. *Arch. Gen. Psychiatry* 22:72–77, 1970.

Berens, S. C., Bernstein, R. S., Robbins, J., and Wolff, J. Antithyroid effects of lithium. *J. Clin. Invest.* 49:1357–1367, 1970.

Branchey, M. H., Charles, J., and Simpson, G. M. Extrapyramidal side effects of lithium maintenance therapy. *Am. J. Psychiatry* 133:444–445, 1976.

Cade, J. F. J. Lithium salts in the treatment of psychotic excitement. *Med. J. Austr.* 36:349–352, 1949.

Cohen, W. J., and Cohen, N. H. Lithium carbonate, haloperidol and irreversible brain damage. *J. A. M. A.* 230:1283–1287, 1974.

Cooper, T. B. and Simpson, G. M. The 24-hour lithium level as a prognosticator of dosage requirements: a two-year follow-up study. *Am. J. Psychiatry* 133:440–443, 1976.

Coppen, A., Shaw, D. M., Malleson, A., and Costain, R. Mineral metabolism in mania. *Brit. Med. J.* 1:71–75, 1966.

Cundall, R. L., Brooks, P. W., and Murray, L. G. A controlled evaluation of lithium prophylaxis in affective disorders. *Psychol. Med.* 2:308–311, 1972.

Davis, J. M. Overview: Maintenance therapy in psychiatry. II. Affective disorders. *Am. J. Psychiatry* 133:1–13, 1976.

Davis, J. M., and Fann, W. E. Lithium. *Ann. Rev. Pharmacol.* 11:285–302, 1971.

Demers, R. G., and Heninger, G. R. Electrocardiographic T-wave changes during lithium carbonate treatment. *J. A. M. A.* 218:381–386, 1971.

Gattozzi, A. A. *Lithium in the Treatment of Mood Disorders,* U. S. National Clearinghouse for Mental Health Information (NIMH), Publication No. 5033. U. S. Government Printing Office, Washington, D. C., 1970.

Gershon, S. Lithium in mania. *Clin. Pharmacol. Ther.* 11:168–187, 1970.

Gershon, S., and Shopsin, B. *Lithium: Its Role in Psychiatric Research and Treatment.* Plenum Press, New York, 1975.

Goldfield, M., and Weinstein, M. R. Lithium in pregnancy: a review with recommendations. *Am. J. Psychiatry* 127:888–893, 1971.

Goldfield, M. D., and Weinstein, M. R. Lithium carbonate in obstetrics: Guidelines for clinical use. *Am. J. Obstet. Gynecol.* 116:15–22, 1973.

Goodwin, F. K., Murphy, D. L., and Bunney, W. E., Jr. Lithium in depression and mania: a double-blind behavioral and biochemical study. *Arch. Gen. Psychiatry* 21:486–496, 1969.

Grof, P., Schou, M., Angst, J., Baastrup, P. C., and Weis, P. Methodological problems of prophylactic trials in recurrent affective disorders. *Brit. J. Psychiatry* 116:599–619, 1970.

Johnson, F. N., ed. *Lithium Research and Therapy.* Academic Press, New York, 1975.

Johnson, G., Gershon, S., Burdock, E. I., et al. Comparative effects of lithium and chlorpromazine in the treatment of acute manic states. *Brit. J. Psychiatry* 119:267–276, 1971.

Kukopulos, A., Reginaldi, D., Girardi, P., and Tondo, L. Course of manic-depressive recurrences under lithium. *Compr. Psychiatry* 16:517–524, 1975.

Mendels, J. Lithium in the treatment of depression. *Am. J. Psychiatry* 133:373–378, 1976.

Neil, J. F., Himmelhoch, J. M., and Licata, S. M. Emergence of myasthenia gravis during treatment with lithium carbonate. *Arch. Gen. Psychiatry* 33:1090–1092, 1976.

Prien, R. F., Caffey, E. M., Jr., and Klett, C. J. A comparison of lithium carbonate and chlorpromazine in the treatment of mania. V. A. Cooperative Studies in Psychiatry: Prepublication report No. 86, Central Neuropsychiatric Research Lab, Perry Point V. A. Hosital, Maryland, 1971.

Prien, R. F., Caffey, E. M., Jr., and Klett, C. J. The relationship between serum lithium level and clinical response in acute manics treated with lithium carbonate. *Brit. J. Psychiatry* 120:409–414, 1972.

Prien, R. F., Caffey, E. M., Jr., and Klett, C. J. Prophylactic efficacy of lithium carbonate in manic-depressive illness. *Arch. Gen. Psychiatry* 28:337–341, 1973.

Prien, R. F., Klett, C. J., and Caffey, E. M., Jr. Lithium carbonate and imipramine in prevention of affective episodes. *Arch. Gen. Psychiatry* 29:420–425, 1973.

Quitkin, F., Rifkin, A., Klein, D. F., and Davis, J. M. On prophylaxis in unipolar depressive disorder. *Am. J. Psychiatry* 133: 1091–1092, 1976.

Quitkin, F., Rifkin, A., and Klein, D. F. Prophylaxis of affective disorders. *Arch. Gen. Psychiatry* 33:337–341, 1976.

Rifkin, A., Kurtin, S. B., Quitkin, F., and Klein, D. F. Lithium-induced folliculitis. *Am. J. Psychiatry* 130:1018–1019, 1973.

Rifkin, A., Quitkin, F., Carrillo, C., et al. Lithium carbonate in emotionally unstable character disorders. *Arch. Gen. Psychiatry* 27:519–523, 1972.

Schou, M. Biology and pharmacology of the lithium ion. *Pharmacol. Rev.* 9:17–58, 1957.

Schou, M. Lithium in psychiatric therapy and prophylaxis. *J. Psychiatr. Res.* 6:67–95, 1968.

Schou, M. The biology and pharmacology of lithium: a bibliography. *NIMH Psychopharmacol. Bull.* 5:33–62, 1969.

Schou, M., Amdisen, A., and Steenstrup, O. R. Lithium and pregnancy. II. Hazards to women given lithium during pregnancy and delivery. *Brit. Med. J.* 2:137–138, 1973.

Schou, M., Amdisen, A. and Trap-Jensen, J. Lithium poisoning. *Am. J. Psychiatry* 125:520–527, 1968.

Shopsin, B., Kim, S. S., and Gershon, S. A controlled study of lithium vs. chlorpromazine in acute schizophrenics. *Brit. J. Psychiatry* 119:435–440, 1971.

Stallone, F., Shelley, E., Mendelwicz, J., and Fieve, R. R. The use of lithium in affective disorders, III: A double blind study of prophylaxis in bipolar illness. *Am. J. Psychiatry* 130:1006–1010, 1973.

Stokes, P. E., Kocsis, J. H., and Arcuni, O. J. Relationship of lithium chloride to treatment response in acute mania. *Arch. Gen. Psychiatry* 33:1080–1084, 1976.

Van der Velde, C. D. Toxicity of lithium carbonate in elderly patients. *Am. J. Psychiatry* 127:1075–1077, 1971.

Vinarova, E., Uhlif, O., Stika, L., and Vinar, O. Side effects of lithium administration. *Act. Nerv. Super.* (Praha) 14:105–107, 1972.

Wilson, J. H. P., Donker, A. J. M., Van Der Hem., G. K., and Wientjes, J. Peritoneal dialysis for lithium poisoning. *Brit. Med. J.* 2:749–750, 1971.

Woody, J. N., London, W. L., and Wilbands, G. D., Jr. Lithium toxicity in a newborn. *Pediatrics* 47:94–96, 1971.

Antidepressant Agents

Alexanderson, B., and Sjoqvist, F. Individual differences in the pharmacokinetics of monomethylated tricyclic antidepressants: role of genetic and environmental factors and clinical importance. *Ann. N. Y. Acad. Sci.* 179:739–751, 1971.

Appel, P., Eckel, K., and Harrer, G. Veränderungen des Blasen- and Blasensphinktertonus durch Thymoleptika: Zystomanometrische Untersuchungen beim Menschen. *Int. Pharmacopsychiatry* 6:15–16, 1971.

Åsberg, M. Plasma nortriptyline levels—relationship to clinical effects. *Clin. Pharmacol. Ther.* 16:215–229, 1974.

Åsberg, M., Cronholm, B., Sjoqvist, F., and Tuck, D. Relationship between plasma levels and therapeutic effect of nortriptyline. *Brit. Med. J.* 3:331–334, 1971.

Ayd, F. J. Long-term administration of doxepin (Sinequan). *Dis. Nerv. Syst.* 32:617–622, 1971.

Berger, F. M. Depression and antidepressant drugs. *Clin. Pharmacol. Ther.* 18:241–248, 1975.

Bickel, M. H., and Weder, H. J. The total fate of a drug. Kinetics of distribution, excretion, and formation of 14 metabolites in rats treated with imipramine. *Arch. Int. Pharmacodyn. Ther.* 173:433–440, 1968.

Bopp, B., and Biel, J. H. Antidepressant drugs. *Life Sci.* 14:415–423, 1974.

Boston Collaborative Drug Surveillance Program: Adverse reactions to the tricyclic-antidepressant drugs. *Lancet* 1:529–531, 1972.

Brackenridge, R. G. Cardiotoxicity of amitriptyline. *Lancet* 2:929–930, 1972.

Braithwaite, R. A., Goulding, R., Theano, G., et al. Plasma concentration of amitriptyline and clinical response. *Lancet* 1:1297–1300, 1972.

Brown, D., Winsberg, B. G., Bialer, I., and Press, M. Imipramine therapy and seizures: Three children treated for hyperactive behavior disorders. *Am. J. Psychiatry* 130:210–212, 1973.

Cole, J. O., and Davis, J. M. Antidepressant drugs. In *Comprehensive Textbook of Psychiatry II*. Freedman, A. M., Kaplan, H. I., and Sadock, B. J., eds. Williams and Wilkins, Baltimore, 1975, pp. 1941–1956.

Couch, J. R., Ziegler, D. K., and Hassanein, R. Amitriptyline in the prophylaxis of migraine. *Neurology* 26:121–127, 1976.

Couper-Smartt, J. D., and Rodham, R. A technique for surveying side-effects of tricyclic drugs with reference to reported sexual effects. *J. Int. Med. Res.* 1:473–476, 1973.

Crombie, D. L., Pinsent, R. J., and Fleming, D. Imipramine in pregnancy. *Brit. Med. J.* 1:745–746, 1972.

Davies, R. K., Tucker, G. J., Harrow, M., and Detre, T. P. Confusional episodes and antidepressant medication. *Am. J. Psychiatry* 128:95–99, 1971.

Eggermont, E., Raveschot, J., Deneve, V., and Casteels-Van Daele, M. The adverse influence of imipramine on the adaptation of the newborn infant to extrauterine life. *Acta Paediat. Belg.* 26:197–204, 1972.

Everett, H. C. The use of bethanechol chloride with tricyclic antidepressants. *Am. J. Psychiatry* 132:1202–1204, 1975.

Fawcett, J., Maas, J. W., and Dekirmenjian, H. Depression and MHPG excretion: response to dextroamphetamine and tricyclic antidepressants. *Arch. Gen. Psychiatry* 26:246–251, 1972.

Feighner, J. P., King, L. F., Schuckit, M. A., et al. Hormonal potentiation of imipramine and ECT in primary depression. *Am. J. Psychiatry* 128:1230–1238, 1972.

Fischbach, R. Die vegetativen Effekte der Antidepressiva im Bereich des Gastro-Intestinaltraktes. *Wien. Med. Wochenschr.* 123 (Suppl. 5): 3–26, 1973.

Flemenbaum, A. Pavor nocturnus: a complication of single daily tricyclic or neuroleptic dosage. *Am. J. Psychiatry* 133:570–572, 1976.

Freeman, J. W., Mundy, G. R., Beattie, R. R., and Ryan, C. Cardiac abnormalities in poisoning with tricyclic antidepressants. *Brit. Med. J.* 2:610–611, 1969.

Frommer, E. A. Treatment in childhood depression with antidepressant drugs. *Brit. Med. J.* 1:729–732, 1967.

Gittelman-Klein, R. and Klein, D. F. School phobia: diagnostic considerations in the light of imipramine effects. *J. Nerv. Ment. Dis.* 156:199–215, 1973.

Glassman, A. H., and Perel, J. M. The clinical pharmacology of imipramine. *Arch. Gen. Psychiatry* 28:649–653, 1973.

Granacher, R. P., and Baldessarini, R. J. Physostigmine: its use in acute anticholinergic syndrome with antidepressant and antiparkinson drugs. *Arch. Gen. Psychiatry* 32:375–380, 1975.

Greenblatt, M., Grosser, G. H. and Wechsler, H. A comparative study of selected antidepressant medications and EST. *Am. J. Psychiatry* 119:144–153, 1962.

Grof, P., and Vinar, O. Maintenance and prophylactic imipramine doses in recurrent depressions. *Activ. Nerv. Sup.* (Praha) 8:383–385, 1966.

Gruvstad, M. Plasma levels of antidepressants and clinical response. *Lancet* 1:95–96, 1973.

Gyermek, L. The pharmacology of imipramine and related antidepressants. *Int. Rev. Neurobiol.* 9:95–115, 1966.

Hoehn, R., Gross, M., and Lasagna, L. A double-blind comparison of placebo and imipramine in the treatment of depressed patients in a state hospital. *J. Psychiatr. Res.* 1:76–91, 1961.

Hoenig, J., and Visram, S. Amitriptyline vs. imipramine in depressive psychoses. *Brit. J. Psychiatry* 110:840–845, 1964.

Holinger, P. C., and Klawans, H. L. Reversal of tricyclic-overdosage-induced central anticholinergic syndrome by physostigmine. *Am. J. Psychiatry* 133:1018–1023, 1976.

Hollister, L., and Overall, J. Reflections on the specificity of action of antidepressants. *Psychosomatics* 6:361–365, 1965.

Hollister, L., Overall, J., Shelton, J., et al. Drug therapy of depression: Amitriptyline, perphenazine, and their combination in different syndromes. *Arch. Gen. Psychiatry* 17:486–493, 1967.

Huessy, H. R., and Wright, A. L. The use of imipramine in children's behavior disorders. *Acta Paedopsychiatr.* (Basel) 37:194–199, 1970.

Idanpaan-Heikkila, J., and Saxen, L. Possible teratogenicity of imipramine and chlorimipramine. *Lancet* 2:282–284, 1973.

Kantor, S. J., Bigger, J. T., Jr., Glassman, A. H., et al. Imipramine-induced heart block. *J. A. M. A.* 231:1364–1366, 1975.

Kessel, A. and Holt, N. F. Depression—an analysis of follow-up study. *Brit. J. Psychiatry* 3:1143–1153, 1965.

Keup, W., Apolito, A., Olinger, L., et al. Tofranil (imipramine) in the treatment of depressive states. *J. Nerv. Ment. Dis.* 130:146–150, 1960.

Kiloh, L., Ball, J., and Garside, R. F. Prognostic factors in treatment of depressive states with imipramine. *Brit. Med. J.* 1:1225–1227, 1962.

Klein, D. F., and Fink, M. Psychiatric reaction patterns to imipramine. *Am. J. Psychiatry* 119:432–438, 1962.

Klerman, G. F., and Cole, J. O. Clinical pharmacology of imipramine and related antidepressant compounds. *Pharmacol. Rev.* 17:101–141, 1965.

Kline, N. S. Antidepressant medications. *J. A. M. A.* 227:1158–1160, 1974.

Kragh-Sorenson, P., Åsberg, M., and Eggert-Hansen, C. Plasma nortriptyline levels in endogenous depression. *Lancet* 1:113–115, 1973.

Krakowski, A. J. Amitriptyline in treatment of hyperkinetic children: a double-blind study. *Psychosomatics* 6:355–360, 1965.

Kuenssberg, E. V. and Knox, J. D. E. Imipramine in pregnancy. *Brit. Med. J.* 2:292–293, 1972.

Kuhn, R. The treatment of depressive states with imipramine hydrochloride. *Am. J. Psychiatry* 115:459–464, 1958.

Lambert, P. A. Les effets indesirables des antidepresseurs tricycliques. *Thérapie* (Paris) 28:269–305, 1973.

Lehmann, H. E., Cohn, C. H., and De Verteuil, R. L. The treatment of depressive conditions with imipramine (G22355). *Canad. Psychiatr. Assoc. J.* 3:155–160, 1958.

Loo, H., and Bousser, M. G. Incidents et accidents des chimiothérapies par les antidepresseurs. *Cah. Méd.* (Paris) 13:777–794, 1972.

Maas, J. W., Fawcett, J. A., and Dekirmenjian, H. Catecholamine metabolism, depressive illness and drug response. *Arch. Gen. Psychiatry* 26:252–262, 1972.

McBride, N. G., and Morrow, A. W. Limb deformities associated with iminodibenzyl hydrochloride. *Med. J. Austr.* 1:492 and 831, 1972.

Malitz, S., and Kanzler, M.: Are antidepressants better than placebo? *Am. J. Psychiatry* 127:1605–1611, 1971.

Moir, D. C. Tricyclic antidepressants and cardiac disease. *Am. Heart J.* 84:841–842, 1973.

Moir, D. C., Dingwall-Fordyce, I., and Weir, R. D. Medicines evaluation and monitoring group: a follow-up study of cardiac patients receiving amitriptyline. *Eur. J. Clin. Pharmacol.* 6:98–101, 1973.

Moody, J., Tait, A., and Todrick, A. Plasma levels of imipramine and desmethylimipramine during therapy. *Brit. J. Psychiatry* 113:183–193, 1967.

Morgan, M. H., and Read, A. E. Antidepressants and liver disease. *Gut* 13:697–701, 1972.

Morris, J. B., and Beck, A. T. The efficacy of antidepressant drugs. *Arch. Gen. Psychiatry* 30:667–674, 1974.

Noble, J., and Matthew, H. Acute poisoning by tricyclic antidepressants: Clinical features and management of 100 patients. *Clin. Toxicol.* 2:403–421, 1969.

Nouri, A., and Cuendet, J. F. Atteintes oculaires au cours des traitements aux thymoleptiques. *Schweiz. Med. Wochenschr.* 101:1178–1180, 1971.

Overall, J. E. and Hollister, L. E. Indications for tricyclic antidepressant drugs. *Dis. Nerv. Syst.* 32:759–763, 1971.

Page, J. G., Bernstein, J. E., Janicki, R. S., and Michelli, F. A. A multi-clinic trial of pemoline in childhood hyperkinesis. In *Clinical Use of Stimulant Drugs in Children,* Conners, C. K., ed. Excerpta Medica, The Hague, 1974.

Petersen, K. E., Andersen, O. O., and Hansen, T. Mode of action and relative value of imipramine and similar drugs in the treatment of nocturnal enuresis. *Eur. J. Clin. Pharmacol.* 7:187–194, 1974.

Pond, S. M., Graham, G. G., Birkett, D. J., and Wade, D. N. Effects of tricyclic antidepressants on drug metabolism. *Clin. Pharmacol. Ther.* 18:191–199, 1975.

Post, R. M., Kotin, J., and Goodwin, F. K. The effects of cocaine on depressed patients. *Am. J. Psychiatry* 131:511–517, 1974.

Poussaint, A. F., and Ditman, K. S. A controlled study of imipramine (Tofranil) in the treatment of childhood enuresis. *J. Pediatr.* 67:283–290, 1965.

Raisfeld, I. H. Cardiovascular complications of antidepressant therapy. Interactions at the adrenergic neuron. *Am. Heart J.* 83:129–133, 1972.

Rasmussen, J. Poisoning with amitriptyline, imipramine and nortriptyline. *Dan. Med. Bull.* 16:201–203, 1966.

Rickels, K., Chung, H. R., Feldman, H. S., et al. Amitriptyline, diazepam and phenobarbital sodium in depressed outpatients. *J. Nerv. Ment. Dis.* 157:442–451, 1973.

Rickels, K., Ward, C., and Schut, L. Different populations, different drug responses—a comparative study of two antidepressants, each used in two different patient groups. *Am. J. Med. Sci.* 247:328–335, 1964.

Saraf, K., and Klein, D. F. The safety of a single daily dose schedule for imipramine. *Am. J. Psychiatry* 128:483–484, 1971.

Sathananthan, G. L., and Gershon, S. Imipramine withdrawal: An akathisia-like syndrome. *Am. J. Psychiatry* 130:1286–1287, 1973.

Sathananthan, G. L., Gershon, S., Almeida, M., et al. Correlation between plasma and cerebrospinal fluid levels of imipramine. *Arch. Gen. Psychiatry* 33:1109–1110, 1976.

Schildkraut, J. J. Norepinephrine metabolites as biochemical criteria for classifying depressive disorders and predicting responses to treatment: Preliminary findings. *Am. J. Psychiatry* 130:695–699, 1973.

Simpson, G. M., Amin, M., Angus, J. W. S., et al. Role of antidepressants and neuroleptics in the treatment of depression. *Arch. Gen. Psychiatry* 27:337–345, 1972.

Simpson, G. M., Lee, J. H., Cuculic, Z., and Kellner, R. Two dosages of imipramine in hospitalized endogenous and neurotic depressives. *Arch. Gen. Psychiatry* 33:1093–1102, 1976.

Skarbek, A. and Smedberg, D. Amitriptyline: a controlled trial in chronic depressive states. *J. Ment. Sci.* 108:859–861, 1962.

Snyder, S., and Yamamura, H. Antidepressants and the muscarinic acetylcholine receptor. *Arch. Gen. Psychiatry* 34:236–239, 1977.

Uhlenhuth, E. H., and Park, L. C. The influence of medication (imipramine) and doctor in relieving depressed psychoneurotic outpatients. *J. Psychiatr. Res.* 2:101–122, 1964.

Waizer, J., Hoffman, S. P., Polizos, P., and Engelhardt, D. M. Outpatient treatment of hyperactive school children with imipramine. *Am. J. Psychiatry* 131:587–591, 1974.

Walter, C. J. S. Clinical significance of plasma imipramine levels. *Proc. R. Soc. Med.* 64:282–285, 1971.

Wharton, R. N., Perel, J. M., Dayton, P. G., and Malitz, S. A potential clinical use for methylphenidate with tricyclic antidepressants. *Am. J. Psychiatry* 127:1619–1625, 1971.

Williams, R. B., and Sherter, C. Cardiac complications of tricyclic antidepressant therapy. *Ann. Intern. Med.* 74:395–398, 1971.

Wilson, I. C., Prange, A. J., McClane, T. K., et al. Thyroid hormone enhancement of imipramine in non-retarded depressions. *N. Engl. J. Med.* 282:1063–1067, 1970.

Winsberg, B. G., Goldstein, S., Yepes, L. E., and Perel, J. M. Imipramine and electrocardiographic abnormalities in hyperactive children. *Am. J. Psychiatry* 132:542–545, 1975.

Wittenborn, J., Plante, M., Burgess, F., and Maurer, H. Comparison of imipramine, ECT, and placebo in the treatment of depression. *J. Nerv. Ment. Dis.* 135:131–137, 1962.

Zeidenberg, P., Perel, J. M., Kanzler, M., et al. Clinical and metabolic studies with imipramine in man. *Am. J. Psychiatry* 127:1321–1326, 1971.

Zung, W. Effect of antidepressant drugs on sleeping and dreaming. Proceedings of the IV World Congress of Psychiatry, Madrid. In *Excerpta Medica, International Congress Series,* No. 150, 1966 pp. 1804–1826.

MAO Inhibitors and Stimulants

Atkinson, R. M., and Ditman, K. S. Tranylcypromine: A review. *Clin. Pharmacol. Ther.* 6:631–655, 1965.

Ayd, F., ed. Combined tricyclic-MAO antidepressant therapy. *Int. Drug Ther. Newsletter* 10:5–7, 1975.

Baldessarini, R. J. Pharmacology of amphetamines. *Pediatrics* 49:694–701, 1972.

Barsa, J., and Sanders, J. C. A comparative study of tranylcypromine and pargyline. *Psychopharmacologia* 6:295–298, 1964.

Bender, L., and Cottington, F. The use of amphetamine sulfate (benzedrine) in child psychiatry. *Am. J. Psychiatry* 99:116–121, 1942.

Blackwell, B., Marley, E., Price, J., and Taylor, D. Hypertensive interactions between monoamine-oxidase inhibitors. *Brit. J. Psychiatry* 113:349–365, 1967.

Bloch, R., Dooneieff, A., Buchberg, A., and Spellman, S. The clinical effects of isoniazid and iproniazid in the treatment of pulmonary tuberculosis. *Ann. Intern. Med.* 40:881–900, 1954.

Bradley, C.: The behavior of children receiving benzedrine. *Am. J. Psychiatry* 94:577–585, 1937.

Bradley, C., and Bowen, M. Amphetamine (benzedrine) therapy of children's behavior disorders. *Am. J. Orthopsychiatry* 11:92–103, 1941.

Conners, C. K. Psychological effects of stimulant drugs in children with minimal brain dysfunction. *Pediatrics* 49:702–708, 1972.

Conners, C. K., Rothschild, G., Eisenberg, L., et al. Dextroamphetamine sulfate in children with learning disorders. *Arch. Gen. Psychiatry* 21:182–190, 1969.

Conners, C. K., Taylor, E., Meo, G., et al. Magnesium pemoline and dextroamphetamine: A controlled study in children with minimal brain dysfunction. *Psychopharmacologia* 26:321–336, 1972.

Crane, G. E. Iproniazid (Marsilid) phosphate, a therapeutic agent for mental disorders and debilitating disease. *Psychiatr. Res. Rep.* 8:142–152, 1957.

Davies, B. E. A pilot study of nialamide at Cambridge. *J. Soc. Genet. Med.* 123:163–172, 1959.

Denckla, M. B., Bemporad, J. R., and MacKay, M. C. Tics following methylphenidate administration: A report of 20 cases. *J. A. M. A.* 235:1349–1351, 1976.

Evans, D., Davison, K., and Pratt, R. The influence of acetylator phenotype on the effect of treating depression with phenelzine. *Clin. Pharmacol. Ther.* 6:430–435, 1965.

Freeman, R. D. Drug effects on learning in children: a selective review of the past thirty years. *J. Special Ed.* 1:17–44, 1966.

Gilbert, J., Donnelly, K. J., Zimmer, L. E., and Kubis, J. F. Effect of magnesium pemoline and methylphenidate on memory improvement and mood in normal aging subjects. *Aging Hum. Devel.* 4:35–51, 1973.

Guilleminault, C., Wilson, R. A., and Dement, W. C. A study on cataplexy. *Arch. Neurol.* 31:225–261, 1974.

Johnstone, E. C., and Marsh, W. Acetylator status and response to phenelzine in depressed patients. *Lancet* 1:567–570, 1973.

Kelly, D., Guirguis, W., Frommer, E., et al. Treatment of phobic states with antidepressants. *Brit. J. Psychiatry* 116:387–398, 1970.

O'Malley, J. E., and Eisenberg, L. The hyperkinetic syndrome. *Semin. Psychiatry* 5:95–103, 1973.

Overall, J. E., Hollister, L. E., Shelton, J., et al. Tranylcypromine compared with dextroamphetamine in hospitalized depressed patients. *Dis. Nerv. Syst.* 27:653–658, 1966.

Pollitt, J. and Young, J. Anxiety state or masked depression? A study based on the action of monoamine oxidase inhibitors. *Brit. J. Psychiatry* 119:143–149, 1971.

Rao, D. B., and Norris, J. R. A double-blind investigation of Hydergine in the treatment of cerebrovascular insufficiency in the elderly. *Johns Hopkins Med. J.* 130:317–324, 1972.

Rapoport, J. L., Quinn, P. O., Bradbard, G., et al. Imipramine and methylphenidate treatments of hyperactive boys. *Arch. Gen. Psychiatry* 30:789–793, 1974.

Raskin, A. Adverse reactions to phenelzine: Results of a nine-hospital depression study. *J. Clin. Pharmacol.* 12:22–25, 1972.

Safer, D. J., and Allen, R. P. Factors influencing the suppressant effects of two stimulant drugs on the growth of hyperactive children. *Pediatrics* 51:660–667, 1973.

Satterfield, J. H., Cantwell, D., Saul, R. E., et al. Response to stimulant drug treatment in hyperactive children: prediction from EEG and neurological findings. *J. Autism Child. Schizo.* 3:36–48, 1973.

Sethna, E. R. A study of refractory cases of depressive illness and their response to combined antidepressant therapy. *Brit. J. Psychiat.* 124:265–272, 1974.

Sjoqvist, F. Interaction between monoamine oxidase (MAO) inhibitors and other substances. *Proc. R. Soc. Med.* 58:967–978, 1965.

Sleator, E. K., Von Neumann, A., and Sprague, R. L. Hyperactive children: a continuous long-term placebo-controlled follow-up. *J. A. M. A.* 229:316–317, 1974.

Spiker, D. G. and Pugh, D. D. Combining tricyclic and monoamine oxidase inhibitor antidepressants. *Arch. Gen. Psychiatry* 33:828–830, 1976.

Solyon, L., Heseltine, G. F. D., McClure, D. J., et al. Behavior therapy vs. drug therapy in the treatment of phobic neurosis. *Canad. Psychiatr. Assoc. J.* 18:25–31, 1973.

Sprague, R. L., and Sleator, E. K. Effects of psychopharmacologic agents on learning disorders. *Pediat. Clin. North Am.* 20:719–735, 1973.

Stockley, I. H. Monoamine oxidase inhibitors. I. Interactions with sympathomimetic amines. *Pharmacol. J.* 210:590–594, 1973.

Stotsky, B. A., Cole, J. O., Lu, L. M. and Smiflin, C. A controlled study of the efficacy of pentylenetetrazole in hard-core hospitalized psychogeriatric patients. *Am. J. Psychiatry* 129:387–391, 1972.

Tyrer, P., Candy, J., and Kelly, D. Phenelzine in phobic anxiety: a controlled trial. *Psychol. Med.* 3:120–124, 1973.

Tyrer, P., Candy, J., and Kelly, D. A study of the clinical effects of phenelzine and placebo in the treatment of phobic anxiety. *Psychopharmacologia* 32:237–254, 1973.

Wender, P. H. *Minimal Brain Dysfunction in Children.* Wiley-Interscience, New York, 1971.

Winsberg, B. G., Bialer, I., Kupietz, S., and Tobias, J. Effects of imipramine and dextroamphetamine on behavior of neuropsychiatrically impaired children. *Am. J. Psychiatry* 128:1425–1431, 1972.

Wyatt, R. J., Fram, D. H., Buchbinder, R., and Snyder, F. Treatment of intractable narcolepsy with a monoamine oxidase inhibitor. *N. Engl. J. Med.* 285:987–991, 1971.

Antianxiety Agents

Berger, F. The relation between the pharmacological properties of meprobamate and the clinical usefulness of the drug. In *Psychopharmacology. A Review of Progress: 1957–1967,* Efron, D. H., ed., U. S. Public Health Service Publication No. 1836. U. S. Government Printing Office, Washington, D. C., 1960, pp. 139–152.

Boston Collaborative Drug Surveillance Program. Clinical depression of the central nervous system due to diazepam and chlordiazepoxide in relation to cigarette smoking and age. *N. Engl. J. Med.* 288:277–280, 1973.

Cole, J. O., and Davis, J. M. Minor tranquilizers, sedatives, and hypnotics. In *Comprehensive Textbook of Psychiatry II.* Freedman, A. M., Kaplan, H. I., and Sadock, B. J., eds. Williams and Wilkins, Baltimore, 1975, pp. 1956–1968.

Covi, L., Lipman, R. S., Pattison, J. H., et al. Length of treatment with anxiolytic sedatives and response to their sudden withdrawal. *Acta Psychiatr. Scand.* 49:51–64, 1973.

DiMascio, A., Shader, R. I., and Harmatz, J. Psychotropic drugs and induced hostility. *Psychosomatics* 10:46–47, 1969.

Essig, C. F. Addiction to non-barbiturate sedative and tranquilizing drugs. *Clin. Pharmacol. Ther.* 5:334–343, 1964.

Ewing, J. Non-narcotic addictive agents. In *Comprehensive Textbook of Psychiatry,* Freedman, A., and Kaplan, H., eds. Williams and Wilkins, Baltimore, 1967, pp. 1003–1011.

Garattini, S., Mussini, E., and Randall, L. O., eds. *The Benzodiazepines.* Raven Press, New York, 1973.

Goldstein, B. J., and Brauzer, B. Pharmacological considerations in the treatment of anxiety and depression in medical practice. *Med. Clin. North Amer.* 55:485–494, 1971.

Greenblatt, D. J. and Shader, R. I. *Benzodiazepines in Clinical Practice.* Raven Press, New York, 1974.

Greenblatt, D. J. and Shader, R. I. The clinical choice of sedative-hypnotics. *Ann. Intern. Med.* 77:91–100, 1972.

Hollister, L. E., Matzenbecker, F. P., and Degan, R. O. Withdrawal reactions to chlordiazepoxide ("Librium"). *Psychopharmacologia* 2:63–68, 1961.

Kalant, H., LeBlanc, A. E., and Gibbons, R. J. Tolerance to and dependence on some non-opiate psychotropic drugs. *Pharmacol. Rev.* 23:135–191, 1971.

Kales, A., Allen, C., Scharf, M. B., and Kales, J. D. Hypnotic drugs and their effectiveness: all night EEG studies of insomniac patients. *Arch. Gen. Psychiatry* 23:226–232, 1970.

Kelly, D., Brown, C. C., and Shafter, J. W. A controlled physiological, clinical and psychological evaluation of chlordiazepoxide. *Brit. J. Psychiatry* 115:1387–1392, 1969.

Matthew, H, ed. *Acute Barbiturate Poisoning.* Excerpta Medica, Amsterdam, 1971.

Mishara, B. L., and Kastenbaum, R. Wine in the treatment of long-term geriatric patients in mental institutions. *J. Am. Geriatr. Soc.* 22:88–94, 1974.

Taylor, R. L., Maurer, J. I., and Tinklenberg, J. R. Management of "bad trips" in an evolving drug scene. *J. A. M. A.* 213: 422–425, 1970.

Winstead, D. K., Anderson, A., Eilers, M. K., *et al.* Diazepam on demand: drug-seeking behavior in psychiatric in-patients. *Arch. Gen. Psychiat.* 30:349–351, 1974.

Drug Interactions and Toxicology

Alexander, C. S., and Nino, A. Cardiovascular complications in young patients taking psychotropic drugs. *Am. Heart J.* 78:757–769, 1969.

Ban, T. A. Drug interactions with psychoactive drugs. *Dis. Nerv. Syst.* 36:164–166, 1975.

Boston Collaborative Drug Surveillance Program: Reserpine and breast cancer. *Lancet* 2:669–671, 1974.

Bourne, P. G., ed. *A Treatment Manual for Acute Drug Abuse Emergencies.* National Clearinghouse for Drug Abuse Information, Rockville, Md., 1974.

Breckenridge, A., and Orne, M. Clinical implications of enzyme induction. *Ann. N. Y. Acad. Sci.* 179:421–431, 1971.

Briant, R. H., Reid, J. L., and Dollery, C. T. Interaction between clonidine and desipramine in man. *Brit. Med. J.* 1:522–523, 1973.

Caranasos, G. J., Stewart, R. B., and Cluff, L. E. Drug-induced illness leading to hospitalization. *J. A. M. A.* 228:713–717, 1974.

Cohen, S. N., and Armstrong, M. F. *Drug Interactions: A Handbook for Clinical Use.* Williams and Wilkins, Baltimore, 1974.

Conney, A. H. Pharmacological implications of microsomal enzyme induction. *Pharmacol. Rev.* 19:317–366, 1967.

Davis, J. M., Bartlett, E., and Termini, B. Overdosage of psychotropic drugs: a review. *Dis. Nerv. Syst.* 29:157–164, 246–256, 1968.

Davis, J. M., Sekerke, J., and Janowsky, D. S. Drug interactions involving the drugs of abuse. *Drug Intel. Clin. Pharm.* 8:120–142, 1974.

El-Yousef, M. K., Janowsky, D. S., Davis, J. M., and Sekerke, H. J. Reversal of antiparkinsonian drug toxicity by physostigmine: a controlled study. *Am. J. Psychiatry* 130:141–145, 1973.

Evaluations of Drug Interactions, 2nd edition. American Pharmaceutical Association, Washington, D. C., 1976.

Fann, W. E. Some clinically important interactions of psychotropic drugs. *South. Med. J.* 66:661–665, 1973.

Formiller, M., and Cohon, M. S. Coumarin and indanedione anticoagulants—potentiators and antagonists. *Am. J. Hosp. Pharm.* 26:574–582, 1969.

Garg, S. *Clinical Guide to Undesirable Drug Interactions and Interferences.* Springer, New York, 1973.

Glasscote, R., Sussex, J. N., Jaffe, J. H., et al. *The Treatment of Drug Abuse.* American Psychiatric Association, Washington, D. C., 1972.

Gram, L. F., and Overo, K. F. Drug interaction: Inhibitory effect of neuroleptics on metabolism of tricyclic antidepressants in man. *Brit. Med. J.* 1:463–465, 1972.

Granacher, R. P., and Baldessarini, R. J. The usefulness of physostigmine in neurology and psychiatry. In *Clinical Neuropharmacology,* Klawans, H. L., ed., Vol. 1. Raven Press, New York, 1976. pp. 63–79.

Greenblatt, D. J., and Shader, R. I. Drug abuse and the emergency room physician. *Am. J. Psychiatry* 131:559–562, 1974.

Griffen, J. P., and D'Arcy, P. F. *A Manual of Adverse Drug Interactions.* J. Wright & Sons, Bristol, 1975.

Hansten, P. D. *Drug Interactions,* 3rd edition. Lea & Febiger, Philadelphia, 1975.

Hollister, L. E. Adverse reactions to psychotherapeutic drugs. In *Drug Treatment of Mental Disorders,* Simpson, L. L., Raven Press, New York, 1976, pp. 267–288.

Hurwitz, N. Predisposing factors in adverse reactions to drugs. *Brit. Med. J.* 1:536–539, 1969.

Janowsky, D. S., El-Yousef, M. K., Davis, J. M., and Fann, W. E. Guanethidine antagonism by antipsychotic drugs. *J. Tenn. Med. Assoc.* 65:620–622, 1972.

Jick, H. Drugs—remarkably non-toxic. *N. Engl. J. Med.* 291:824–828, 1974.

Kaufmann, J. S. Drug interactions involving psychotherapeutic agents. In *Drug Treatment of Mental Disorders,* Simpson, L. L., ed. Raven Press, New York, 1976, pp. 289–309.

Kline, N. S., Alexander, S. F., and Chamberlain, A. *Psychotropic Drugs: A Manual for Emergency Management of Overdosage.* Medical Economics, Oradell, N. J., 1974.

Kuntzman, R. Drugs and enzyme induction. *Ann. Rev. Pharmacol.* 9:21–36, 1969.

Lemberger, L. Clinically important antihypertensive drug interactions. *Drug Therapy* 49–55, December 1974.

Lennard, H. L., Epstein, L. J., Bernstein, A., and Ransom, D. C. Hazards implicit in prescribing psychoactive drugs. *Science* 169:438–441, 1970.

Lilienfeld, A. M., Chang, L., Thomas, C. B., and Levin, M. L. Rauwolfia derivatives and breast cancer. *Johns Hopkins Med. J.* 139:41–50, 1975.

Lubran, M. The effects of drugs on laboratory values. *Med. Clin. North Amer.* 53:211–222, 1969.

McDonall, A., Owen, S., and Robin, A. A. A controlled comparison of diazepam and amylobarbitone in anxiety states. *Brit. J. Psychiatry* 112:629–631, 1966.

Mack, T. M., Henderson, B. E., Gerkins, V. R., et al. Reserpine and breast cancer in a retirement community. *N. Engl. J. Med.* 292:1366–1371, 1975.

Marsden, C. D., Tarsy, D., and Baldessarini, R. J. Spontaneous and drug-induced movement disorders in psychiatric patients. In *Psychiatric Aspects of Neurologic Disease,* Benson, D. F., and Blumer, D., eds. Grune and Stratton, New York, 1975, pp. 219–265.

Martin, E. W. *Hazards of Medication.* Lippincott, Philadelphia, 1971.

Miller, R. R. Hospital admissions due to adverse drug reactions: A report from the Boston Collaborative Drug Surveillance Program. *Arch. Intern. Med.* 134:219–223, 1974.

Morrelli, H. F. Rational therapy of drug overdosage. In *Clinical Pharmacology. Basic Principles in Therapeutics.* Goodman, L., and Gilman, A., eds. MacMillan, New York, 1972, pp. 605–623.

Morselli, P. L., Cohen, S. N., and Garattini, S., eds. *Drug Interactions.* Raven Press, New York, 1974.

Nies, A. S. Drug interactions. *Med. Clin. North Amer.* 58:965–975, 1974.

Raisfeld, I. H. Clinical pharmacology of drug interactions. *Ann. Rev. Med.* 24:385–418, 1973.

Raskind, M. A. Psychosis, polydipsia and water intoxication. *Arch. Gen. Psychiatry* 30:112–114, 1974.

Sayers, A. C. and Burki, H. R. Antiacetylcholine activities of psychoactive drugs: A comparison of the $[^3H]$quinuclidinylbenzilate binding assay with conventional methods. *J. Pharm. Pharmacol.* 28:252–253, 1976.

Scientific Review Subpanel on Psychotherapeutic Agents. *Evaluation of Drug Interactions.* American Pharmaceutical Association, Washington, D. C., 1973.

Seidl, L. G., Thornton, F., Smith, J. W., and Cluff, L. E. Studies on the epidemiology of adverse drug reactions. III. Reactions in patients on a general medical service. *Bull. Johns Hopkins Hosp.* 119:229–315, 1966.

Shader, R. I., and DiMascio, A., eds. *Psychotropic Drug Side Ef-*

fects: Clinical and Theoretical Perspectives. Williams and Wilkins, Baltimore, 1970.

Shader, R. I. ed. *Psychiatric Complications of Medical Drugs.* Raven Press, New York, 1972.

Sher, S. P. Drug enzyme induction and drug interactions. Literature tabulation. *Toxicol. Appl. Pharmacol.* 18:780–834, 1973.

Swidler, G. *Handbook of Drug Interactions.* Wiley-Interscience, New York, 1971.

Wilkinson, G. R. Treatment of drug intoxication: A review of some scientific principles. *Clin. Toxicol.* 3:249–265, 1970.

Index